D1566439

SPINAL CORD INJURIES
(PGPS-88)

Related Titles

Catalano   *Health, Behavior and the Community: An Ecological Perspective*

Gatchel/Price   *Clinical Applications of Biofeedback: Appraisal and Status*

Katz/Zlutnick   *Behavior Therapy and Health Care: Principles and Applications*

McDaniel   *Physical Disability and Human Behavior, 2nd Edition*

SPINAL CORD INJURIES

Psychological, Social and Vocational Adjustment

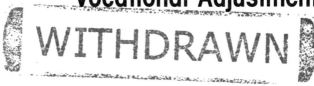

Roberta B. Trieschmann

Director of Psychological Services
St. Jude Hospital and
Rehabilitation Center,
Fullerton, California

Pergamon Press

New York □ Oxford □ Toronto □ Sydney □ Frankfurt □ Paris

Pergamon Press Offices:

U.S.A	Pergamon Press Inc., Maxwell House, Fairview Park, Elmsford, New York 10523, U.S.A.
U.K.	Pergamon Press Ltd., Headington Hill Hall, Oxford OX3 0BW, England
CANADA	Pergamon of Canada Ltd., 150 Consumers Road, Willowdale, Ontario M2J 1P9, Canada
AUSTRALIA	Pergamon Press (Aust) Pty. Ltd., P.O. Box 544, Potts Point, NSW 2011, Australia
FRANCE	Pergamon Press SARL, 24 rue des Ecoles, 75240 Paris, Cedex 05, France
FEDERAL REPUBLIC OF GERMANY	Pergamon Press GmbH, 6242 Kronberg/Taunus, Pferdstrasse 1, Federal Republic of Germany

Library of Congress Cataloging in Publication Data

Trieschmann, Roberta B   1939-
  Spinal cord injuries.

  (Pergamon general psychology series)
  Bibliography: p.
  Includes index.
  1. Spinal cord–Wounds and injuries–Psychological
aspects. 2. Spinal cord–Wounds and injuries–Social
aspects. 3. Paralytics–Rehabilitation. I. Title.
(DNLM: Spinal cord injuries–Psychology. 2. Spinal
cord injuries–Rehabilitation. WL400 T827a)
RD594.3.T74 1979   155.9'16   79-20266
ISBN 0-08-024661-3

Printed in the United States of America

To Clyde

Contents

List of Figures and Tables

Preface

There are few physical disabilities that are as complex and as challenging as spinal cord injury. The psychosocial impact of the disability on a human life has been underestimated and only recently have hospitals and rehabilitation centers been including clinical psychologists and others trained in the behavioral disciplines on the staff. Yet professionals have found that little has been reliably demonstrated about the process of adjustment to severe disability, and myths have been perpetuated without question. Therefore, this book has been written in order to identify what we know and do not know about the process of adjustment to a severe disability—spinal cord injury.

Persons with severe disabilities have much to say about the process of adjustment to such problems. Recently, consumers of rehabilitation services have become more vocal regarding procedures and regulations affecting their daily lives. Yet a large number of professionals do not know what the concerns of the disabled community are because there has been a distance between the professionals and the consumer groups. Therefore, this book has been written with the further intention of imbuing the viewpoints of professionals with the realities of daily life of those with disabilities.

Many people believe that work in the field of physical disability must be depressing because they have a vision of custodial care and of crippled lives filled with sadness and lost dreams. In actuality, rehabilitation of the physically disabled is especially rewarding because of the potential that exists in human beings in the face of stress, a potential that has been seriously underestimated. Physical disabilities occur to our family members, our friends, and our neighbors. Therefore, this book has also been written in order to present a different image of work with the disabled—an image of hope and ample reward for those in many disciplines.

This work should be useful to psychologists, social workers, vocational counselors, physicians, nurses, occupational therapists, physical counselors, physicians, nurses, occupational therapists, physical therapists, and recreational therapists, either as students or practicing professionals. It will serve to dispel myths and to provide a more empirical basis for research and clinical practice. Many questions have been identified and few answers given. Thus, there is an emphasis on the critical evaluation of past literature and research since so much has been uncritically accepted as fact, yet so much needs to be demonstrated as true.

A significant portion of the research for this book was financed by a research grant from the Rehabilitation Services Administration, HEW, to do a state-of-the-art study of the psychological, social, and vocational adjustment to spinal cord injury (Trieschmann 1978a). This project involved an exhaustive review of the literature, an advisory committee, a conference of professionals, and a conference of persons with spinal cord injury. This latter group served as a consumer advisory panel to this author after the project ended and during the writing of this book. They reviewed the manuscript and made suggestions for additions or changes. It is of interest to note that the one feature of this book that they prized the most was the critical evaluation of the literature on adjustment to disability. Apparently, they have felt victimized by professionals who write articles about the reactions to disability that are based more on theory than fact. Thus, if this book serves any purpose, it will be to prompt a moratorium on speculation and theorizing and increase our efforts to provide an empirical basis for our professional activities with the disabled population.

Acknowledgments

There are many individuals and organizations that have provided invaluable assistance during the research and writing of this book. The Easter Seal Society of Los Angeles County provided the fiscal management of the research grant from the Rehabilitation Services Administration, and I am grateful to Alan H. Facter, executive director, and June Taylor, program director, for their kindness and support. J. Paul Thomas of the Rehabilitation Services Administration has provided unlimited support for this endeavor. His encouragement is much appreciated. The advisory committee for the research phase included Theodore M. Cole, M.D., George W. Hohmann, Ph.D., Mary Ann Mikulic, M.N., R.N., Mary Romano, M.S.W., and Carolyn L. Vash, Ph.D. Their help was invaluable in providing structure and advice throughout the research phase. Gary T. Athelstan, Ph.D., David Barrie, Mickey Christiason, M.T.R.S., Wayne Dexter, Ph.D., Wilbert Fordyce, Ph.D., Richard T. Goldberg, Ed.D., Robert Allen Keith, Ph.D., John Marr, Ph.D., and N. Elane Wilcox, Ph.D., provided inputs which were helpful in the formulation of the manuscript.

Particular thanks must be expressed to my consumer advisory panel: Gerald Davis, Glenn Goldmann, Allan Jarabin, Phillip Kaplan, Nancy Becker Kennedy, Polly McBroom, Tad Tanaka, and Sheila Velez. Their interest and time were freely given and without their help this book would have been of little value.

The data contained in figure 1.2 and tables 1.1, 1.2, 1.3, and 1.4 are derived from information contained in the *National Spinal Cord Injury Model Systems Conference: Proceedings* (1978).

My colleagues at St. Jude Hospital and Rehabilitation Center have been extremely patient while I finished the manuscript, and Dr. Francis Mackey, medical director, and my staff, Mrs. Judy Stewart, and Mrs. Billie Martin have been particularly supportive during this trying period. I truly appreciate their understanding and help. Sister Jane Frances, president of the hospital, generously supported this effort and provided the assistance of her secretary, Mrs. Deborah Hlavac, to type a large part of the manuscript. For this I am very grateful, and I must commend Mrs. Hlavac for her consistent cordiality and outstanding secretarial skills.

Throughout the three years of this endeavor, my husband, A. Clyde Flackbert, Ph.D., has lived the experience with me, serving occasionally as typist, xerographer, collator, proofreader, sounding board, critic, and moral supporter. I am deeply grateful for his love and support which have made this effort possible.

Part I
Spinal Cord Injury and the Rehabilitation Process

1

The Consequences of Spinal Cord Injury

A STATEMENT OF THE PROBLEM

Spinal cord injury is a low incidence but high-cost disability that usually requires tremendous changes in the person's style of life. It has been estimated that there are 150,000 persons with spinal injuries in the United States at the present time and that 7,000 to 10,000 new spinal injuries occur each year (National Spinal Cord Injury Model Systems Conference 1978). Approximately 62 percent of the spinal injuries occur to persons aged 15 through 29. Thus, the population is young, and with the advances in medical science, this group may achieve a life expectancy that is not too different from that of the able-bodied person. However, estimates of the lifetime care costs for the average person with quadriplegia are $325,000 to $400,000 (using a conservative estimate of life expectancy of 50 percent less than normal). The lifetime care costs for persons with paraplegia are estimated to be $180,000 to $225,000 (National Spinal Cord Injury Model Systems Conference 1978). As a result, the financial burden imposed upon the person, the family, and the nation is tremendous.

Yet any estimate of the cost of spinal injury must include those intangible issues to which a monetary value cannot be attached. These issues include: the devaluation of the disabled person by society; the frustrations and hard work associated with the daily activities of survival; the stress on family relationships and traditional roles; and the loss of satisfaction from vocational and leisure time activities which may no longer be possible after spinal injury. Thus, it is these issues that become the core of the process of adjustment to spinal injury.

Among the several definitions of the word "adjustment," the *Random House Dictionary* (1973) includes two that are relevant to the topic of this book: "the act of bringing something into conformity with external requirements; harmony achieved by modification or alteration of a position."

The onset of a spinal injury introduces many physical impairments that change the person's ability to carry out activities such as ambulation, grooming, toileting, and many other activities of daily living (ADL). In addition to the physical impairments, there are psychosocial consequences that have a profound impact on the person's perception of himself or herself. Therefore, adjustment is necessary because the external requirements for living suddenly change after spinal injury. However, adjustment, under these circumstances, will be a whole series of acts and, consequently, it is more appropriate to discuss the *process* of adjustment to spinal injury. The goal of this adjustment process will be harmony between the person and his or her new circumstances of life. Yet, harmony is not necessarily synonymous with happiness for able-bodied or disabled persons, and within all of our lives there will be changes, new demands, new stresses to which we must accommodate and adjust, always with the aim of achieving harmony with our own environment. This is a daily process and the degree of harmony that we achieve will vary over time. Thus, it is no different for a newly disabled person. The onset of a spinal injury will place a person in disharmony with many aspects of his or her world, and, therefore, the process of adjustment may be long and complicated, difficult and multifaceted.

THE PHYSICAL SEQUELAE OF SPINAL CORD INJURY

An injury to the spinal cord may produce symptoms that are temporary or permanent and impairment of function that may be incomplete or complete. An incomplete lesion is one in which certain amounts of motor and sensory function below the level of the injury will be intact, whereas a complete lesion is one in which sensory and motor loss is total below the level of the injury. Consequently, the implications for future functioning may be significantly different for two individuals who are injured at the same vertebral level if one has a complete lesion and one has an incomplete lesion.

Motor and sensory function will vary depending upon the level of the injury. Those injuries occurring at the cervical level of the vertebral column (neck) will result in quadriplegia (if complete) or quadriparesis (if incomplete). Injuries occurring in the thoracic, lumbar, or sacral regions of the vertebral column (trunk or low back) will result in paraplegia (if complete) or paraparesis (if incomplete). Figure 1.1 displays the vertebral column and the nerve supply to the body.

In this section, some of the physical impairments and complications of spinal injury will be reviewed briefly. They are: paralysis of motor function, loss of sensation, loss of bladder and bowel control, and an altered ability to participate in the physical parameters of sexual relationship.

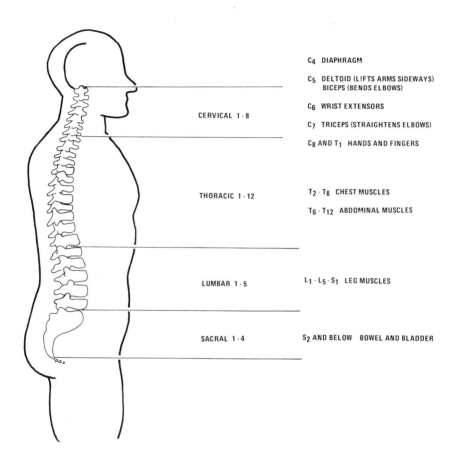

CERVICAL 1 - 8

THORACIC 1 - 12

LUMBAR 1 - 5

SACRAL 1 - 4

C_4 DIAPHRAGM

C_5 DELTOID (LIFTS ARMS SIDEWAYS)
      BICEPS (BENDS ELBOWS)

C_6 WRIST EXTENSORS

C_7 TRICEPS (STRAIGHTENS ELBOWS)

C_8 AND T_1 HANDS AND FINGERS

T_2 - T_8 CHEST MUSCLES

T_6 - T_{12} ABDOMINAL MUSCLES

L_1 - L_5 - S_1 LEG MUSCLES

S_2 AND BELOW BOWEL AND BLADDER

Fig. 1.1. Vertebral column and nerve supply.

Motor Impairment

Quadriplegia. Spinal cord injuries that occur in the cervical region are called quadriplegia and the amount of residual function depends upon the cervical level of the injury. Those injured at C_1 and C_2 will have no motor function below the head and they will be unable to breathe without use of a respirator. They will require total assistance and independent function will be limited to the use of the muscles of the face.

Injuries at C_3 lead to paralysis below the neck but there may be a bit of shoulder function intact. Breathing will be by use of a respirator and the person will require assistance with almost all activities. Individuals with injuries at C_3 and above may be able to use an electric wheelchair, controlled by head movements or shoulder movements, that is equipped with a portable respirator.

Independent respiration is possible for those injured at C_4 since the diaphragm is innervated at this level. However, the upper extremities will be paralyzed and assistance will be needed for almost all activities.

Persons with a C_5 functional level will be able to use their shoulder and biceps which will permit some upper arm mobility. Powered hand splints will provide some hand function and an electric wheelchair will be the mode of locomotion. Assistance with most daily activities will be necessary.

At C_6 the *potential* for independence is present. Because of the ability to extend the wrist, the person might be able to transfer into and out of the wheelchair alone and might be able to carry out many of the other activities of daily living alone. However, finger function will be absent. Independent living may be possible but attainment of such a goal will require much physical effort and time. An electric wheelchair will not be necessary, and the person may be able to drive an automobile with hand controls.

At C_7 independence is definitely probable, although finger dexterity will be markedly impaired. Independent function will be time-consuming and require much energy, but the option is there. At C_8 some finger function is present and, thus, independent living is assured, depending upon the person.

Paraplegia. Spinal injuries in the thoracic, lumbar, and sacral levels will result in paraplegia, paralysis in the lower extremities.

Injuries between T_1 and T_8 will involve paralysis of the chest and trunk muscles, abdominal muscles, and the leg muscles. As a result, balance and trunk stability will be a potential problem and all functions must be managed through shoulder, arm, and hand function alone. A manual wheelchair will be used and independence in all activities is possible.

Injuries at T_9 and below will lead to impaired hip and leg function. Ambulation with long leg braces and crutches may be feasible for those with injuries in the lumbar region although the energy expenditure will be great. Thus, a wheelchair may be the preferred mode of locomotion. Ambulation is definitely possible for those with sacral lesions and only short leg braces may be needed with crutches or canes.

Sensory Impairment

In complete lesions, the area of sensory loss will roughly approximate the area of motor loss although the sensory and motor nerve tracts are different. Thus, below the level of the lesion, there will be a loss of the sense of touch, temperature, pain, and position. The functional implications of this sensory loss are significant since injury can occur to anesthetic parts of the body without the person's awareness.

Care must be taken to avoid burns from water that is too hot or from proximity to a heater. In northern climates, frostbite would be a possibility unless skin temperature was monitored. Pain is a signal that something is wrong. Thus, the absence of pain sensation can be a mixed blessing. The loss of touch and pain sense is an unfortunate combination that predisposes a person with spinal injury to pressure sores (decubitus ulcers).

To adjust and shift position is normal in able-bodied persons; in this way pressure is constantly being relieved and redistributed across skin areas. However, persons with spinal injury do not sense a discomfort which urges them to shift position. Thus, pressure sores are one of the most important complications following spinal injury. A pressure sore is an area of damage to the skin and tissue underneath caused by unrelieved pressure sufficient to interrupt proper circulation. These ulcerations are more likely to occur on underlying bony prominences such as the buttocks and sacral area, heels, ankles, and hips.

Prevention of pressure sores is easier than treatment; thus, persons with spinal injury are taught methods of skin care and position shifting which attempt to reduce the incidence of this complication. Once a pressure sore has been identified, treatment can be lengthy and costly. Pressure must be removed from the area of the decubitus, and this usually disrupts a person's daily activity schedule quite extensively. Surgical intervention may be necessary in severe cases.

Bladder and Bowel Dysfunctions

The onset of a complete spinal injury will result in the loss of voluntary control over bladder and bowel function. Thus, initially an indwelling catheter in the bladder will provide for drainage of the urine. The catheter will be removed and a program of intermittent catheterization initiated as bladder training procedures are instituted. Males will usually eliminate reliance on an indwelling catheter and can use an external urinary collection device or intermittent catheterization. However, there is no acceptable external urinary collection device for females; thus, they usually will continue to use an indwelling catheter. Some rehabilitation programs have a policy of removing all catheters before discharge. Consequently, this may force some women to wear diapers which can be a socially and psychologically devastating situation.

Following spinal injury, there are certain steps that the disabled person must take to maintain a healthy urinary tract system. Much fluid must be consumed each day; the urine should be acidified (through medication or diet); and periodic evaluations of the kidney and bladder should be scheduled. The presence of an indwelling catheter increases the probability of bladder infection, and loss of calcium from the bones increases the chances of kidney and bladder stones. Kidney damage is one of the primary causes of death in those who successfully survive the spinal injury.

A bowel program will be planned in order to train the bowel to empty on schedule. A routine is essential for management of the bowel; therefore, life as a spinal injured person loses much of its flexibility and spontaneity. The bowel can be trained to empty itself every one, two, or three days at morning or evening. Maintenance of a proper diet is essential since certain types of food can disrupt the bowel schedule. Thus, socially embarrassing accidents can be avoided by attention to diet and bowel schedule.

Sexual Function

The degree and type of sexual dysfunction following spinal injury depends upon the sex of the individual, the level of the lesion, and the completeness of the injury.

Among females with spinal injury, the motor paralysis need not be a deterrent to participation in sexual acts, but the lack of sensation may alter the degree of pleasure experienced. In complete spinal injuries, there will be no sensation of orgasm, but there may be other subtle physiological signs of an orgasmlike state (Griffith and Trieschmann 1976). Many women experience considerable pleasure from participation in sexual acts because of the emotional relationship with the partner and some learn to experience phantom orgasm (Bregman and Hadley 1976). We do not have much information about the stages of physiological sexual arousal in spinal injured women, but we do know that fertility is unimpaired. Menstrual periods tend to resume within several months of the spinal injury. In incomplete spinal injuries, the woman has an increased probability of experiencing the entire range of sexual pleasures. However, sexual pleasure is always the result of a combination of physical and psychological factors.

Males with spinal injury will experience disruption of sexual acts because of their motor paralysis and sensory deficit. In addition, there will often be an interference in the ability to obtain an erection. Level of injury and completeness of the lesion will be the key factor in the ability to have erections.

Nondisabled males experience erections on a psychogenic basis. That is, in response to a sexual stimulus, one sign of male arousal is an erection. In complete spinal injuries, erections do not occur to a sexual stimulus. If they occur, it is by spinal reflex and, therefore, they are not on a voluntary basis and are not psychologically related to a sexual situation. Males with complete spinal injuries in the cervical and thoracic areas will experience reflexogenic erections. Tactile pressure in the genital area, rubbing of the penis, pulling of hairs in the genital area, pulling on the catheter may be ways of triggering the reflex erection. Males with complete spinal injuries in the lumbar and sacral areas will not be able to obtain any erection, even on a reflex basis. With incomplete spinal injuries, the probability of psychogenic erections increases significantly, including those injured in the lumbar and sacral regions.

Although erections may occur on a reflex basis, sexual intercourse is possible in many cases and the strategies to accomplish this depend upon the preferences of the partners. Mooney, Cole, and Chilgren (1975) and Griffith and Trieschmann (1976) should be consulted for more information.

Fertility in males with spinal injury is usually impaired since ejaculations may not occur. When ejaculations do occur, the semen is ejected into the bladder rather than out of the penis which effectively precludes conception in most cases. Artificial insemination is a possibility that couples should explore following a spinal injury.

Despite the physical interference with sexual function, many men have satisfying sexual experiences with their partners (Berkman, Weissman, and Frielich 1978). As with spinal injured females with complete lesions, phantom orgasm is a possibility, and much satisfaction can be derived from a partner's pleasure. In chapter 6, the issue of sexuality will be discussed in all of its dimensions, the psychosocial aspects in particular.

Further Complications of Spinal Cord Injury

There are several other factors that need to be considered when describing the physical consequences of spinal cord injury. The issues of pain, muscle spasm, autonomic dysreflexia, temperature regulation, and respiratory function may have a significant impact on the person's daily life depending on the level and circumstances of the injury.

Pain. The trauma that results in damage to the spinal cord will usually be significant and ordinarily leads to pain at the level of the injury. In complete spinal injuries, there will be anesthesia below the level of the lesion, but at the lesion, pain may be a problem for a couple of weeks. Usually, however, this pain will not be a problem over time unless there have been multiple surgeries with scarring (Burke 1973). Spinal injuries resulting from gunshot wounds often tend to be associated with pain for longer periods of time, perhaps because of the scarring along the pathway of the bullet.

Parathesias and hypesthesias may be a source of discomfort to some persons with spinal injuries. Parathesias are unusual sensations, such as a burning or tingling, along nerve roots which the person may label as pain. In many cases these sensations disappear with time. In the author's experience, hypnosis provides only temporary relief in these situations, and the posthypnotic suggestion of relief from discomfort needs to be reinforced every three to four days. Hypesthesias is an increased sensitivity over certain areas of the body, which may or may not be discomforting to the person. There is often an increased sensitivity at or just below the sensory level of the lesion which can be a source of erotic stimulation during sexual encounters.

Muscle Spasms. Immediately after the spinal injury, there will be a state of spinal shock during which there will be an absence of all reflexes below the level of the injury. Over a period of months, however, reflexes will return to those whose injuries are in the cervical and thoracic regions. In certain individuals, there may be exaggerated somatic reflexes which lead to muscle activity of a reflexive, nonvoluntary nature. In the early stages of the spinal injury, such muscle movement is often misinterpreted as recovery by the person and family and, thus, careful evaluation by the physician is required.

Most persons with spinal injuries in the cervical and thoracic regions will have intermittent muscle spasms which may or may not be noticeable to others. Occasionally, an individual may be plagued by such severe and frequent muscle spasms that surgical or drastic chemotherapeutic intervention may be necessary. Such interventions are considered only when the spasms consistently interfere with the performance of daily activities.

Autonomic Dysreflexia. Autonomic dysreflexia is a pathological reflex in which the person's blood pressure suddenly elevates to dangerously high levels. Unless the blood pressure is reduced rapidly, cerebral hemorrhage may result. This problem tends to occur only in those persons with spinal injuries in the cervical or high thoracic (above $T_4 - T_6$) regions, and some individuals are lucky enough to never experience this problem. Distention of the bladder is the most common cause of this problem. Thus, emptying of the bladder contents is a key intervention strategy. Autonomic dysreflexia which is usually signaled by a pounding headache, sweating of the forehead, goose bumps, and a stuffy nose constitutes a medical emergency, and treatment should be sought immediately.

Temperature regulation. Those with spinal injuries in the cervical and high thoracic (above $T_4 - T_6$) regions also may have trouble with temperature regulation and sweating. An inability to shiver, lack of vasoconstriction to conserve heat in cold climates, and an inability to perspire to vaporize heat in warm climates may make the person quite uncomfortable. Thus, the body temperature will be greatly influenced by the temperature of the external environment. Occasionally, some persons with injuries in this area will experience excessive sweating above the level of the lesion. Those with incomplete lesions may have additional localized sweating below the lesion level. At these times the sweating may drench the area involved and thus be physically uncomfortable and socially embarrassing to the person.

Respiratory function. Individuals with spinal injuries in the cervical and in the high thoracic region will have markedly limited chest expansion during breathing and an inability to cough adequately to remove secretions in the lungs. Breathing will be by the diaphragm for those injured at C_4 and below because the chest muscles are paralyzed. Thus, the person is quite vulnerable to respiratory infections and must be very careful during "cold" or "flu" season. Having a respiratory infection becomes more serious than in the nondisabled population.

THE REHABILITATION PROCESS

Acute Management of the Spinal Cord Injury

Proper treatment of spinal cord injury must begin at the scene of the accident. Persons trained in emergency medical procedures should be summoned, and every effort must be made to immobilize the spine at the site of the accident and during transport to the hospital.

At the acute treatment center, the spinal injury and associated injuries will be assessed. Surgery to stabilize the vertebral column may be necessary, and the person will be immobilized on a specially designed bed, such as a stryker frame for example. Persons with cervical injuries may need to have holes drilled into the skull and tongs inserted so that traction can be maintained upon the neck. Thus, the head will be immobilized along with the rest of the body. Proper respiratory function will be maintained by performance of a tracheostomy and use of a respirator for persons with high cervical injuries. A catheter will be inserted into the bladder to insure adequate drainage of urine and intravenous fluids will be started to maintain a proper fluid and electrolyte balance.

Consequently, in addition to the paralysis induced by the injury, the person is further immobilized by the stryker frame and tubes will be running into and out of the body at various points. Every two hours, around the clock, every day, the stryker frame will be turned and the person will be flipped like a pancake, so to speak, in order to change the pressure on the skin and prevent pressure sores. Thus, the person's visual field will be restricted to the floor and ceiling. Persons with an open tracheostomy cannot vocalize very effectively; thus, communication will be restricted. Everything will have to be done for the person, including scratching an itchy nose for a person with quadriplegia.

When the vertebral column has stabilized and movement is possible without the risk of further injury to the spinal cord, the person will be a well and healthy person, no longer sick, and rehabilitation will swing into full action. This may entail the transfer to a completely different hospital or facility or merely an intensification of activities already initiated if acute care has been received within a specialized spinal cord injury treatment center. However, whether or not there is a physical transfer of the person with spinal injury, rehabilitation ushers in a totally different focus for everyone's efforts.

In the acute stage, medical management of the physical trauma was the focus as most personnel were actively engaged in doing things to and for the person with spinal injury. However, when the injury has healed, the person is left with a physical disability, an inability to perform certain activities because of paralysis and sensory loss. Consequently, the focus must become an educational one with the spinal injured person in the role of the student and the rehabilitation personnel in the role of teacher. This transition in emphasis is not always clearly perceived by the disabled person who may continue to hope that in time he or she will ''get better.'' In addition, the location of rehabilitation activities in a hospital with all of the symbols of treatment and therapy (white uniforms, hospital rooms, therapy areas) tends to obscure this shift in emphasis from one of care to one of education. The operational policies of hospitals further tend to obscure this shift in emphasis by counting units of treatment for accountability purposes. However, units of treatment may not be an appropriate measure when applied to an educational process.

Formal Rehabilitation

During the traditional rehabilitation phase, the person with a spinal injury must learn to perform all of the activities required for survival as an independent adult. If the paralysis is extensive enough, as in high quadriplegia, the person must learn what needs to be done for him or her and learn to arrange for others to do the necessary activities for survival.

Traditionally, rehabilitation has been focused on teaching techniques of mobility and activities of daily living (ADL). Mobility training will include learning to change position in bed, to transfer from the bed to the wheelchair and reverse, to use a wheelchair, to transfer from the wheelchair to a car and reverse, to get the wheelchair into the car, to drive a car with hand controls, and for persons with injuries in the lumbar and sacral regions, ambulation with braces and crutches. Persons trained in physical therapy often take the primary responsibility for mobility training.

ADL training includes such activities as bathing, grooming, getting dressed, skin care, bladder and bowel management, eating, and homemaking skills. These activities are usually taught by persons trained in occupational therapy and nursing. For persons with quadriplegia, ADL training can become one of the primary emphases within rehabilitation because of their limited hand and finger function. Adaptive devices may be made by the occupational therapist which will assist the person in accomplishing certain tasks, such as a tenodesis splint which uses wrist extension to obtain a grasp.

These ADL and mobility skills are taught within a rehabilitation center which may or may not be part of an acute care hospital. Individuals of many disciplines will have contact with the disabled person during this rehabilitation process, such as physicians (usually a physiatrist who is trained in physical medicine and rehabilitation), nurses, psychologists, social workers, vocational counselors, physical therapists, occupational therapists, recreational therapists, orthotists (experts in brace manufacture), and sometimes the biomedical engineer. Therefore, the team approach is customary in rehabilitation and the efficiency of the rehabilitation process will be correlated with the quality of the communication among team members.

When the team determines that the disabled person can perform all of the mobility and ADL tasks of which he or she is capable, discharge to the home environment will be recommended. Ideally, the person's family members will have been actively involved in learning about the disability during the inpatient rehabilitation phase. In any case, the family will be given last minute information and training so that the disabled person's transition to life outside of the hospital will be as smooth as possible.

THE TREATMENT SYSTEMS

The Regional Model Spinal Cord Injury Treatment System

Since 1970, the Rehabilitation Services Administration (RSA) of the Department of Health, Education, and Welfare has sponsored a series of regional model spinal cord injury centers, geographically spaced across the United States to promote the proper management of persons with spinal injury. The systems concept has been demonstrated to reduce the cost of treatment of newly injured persons by preventing complications that may arise as a result of lack of coordination of service delivery (Matlack 1974). As of spring 1979, the regional model spinal cord injury treatment centers were located in the following places:

1. University of Washington Medical Center, Seattle, Washington
2. Santa Clara Valley Medical Center, San Jose, California
3. Good Samaritan Hospital and St. Joseph's Hospital, Phoenix, Arizona
4. Craig Hospital, Denver, Colorado
5. Rehabilitation Institute of Chicago and Northwestern Memorial Hospital, Chicago, Illinois
6. University of Missouri Medical Center, Columbia, Missouri
7. University of Alabama Medical Center, Birmingham, Alabama
8. Institute for Rehabilitation and Research, Houston, Texas
9. University of Miami Medical Center, Miami, Florida
10. Woodrow Wilson Rehabilitation Center and University of Virginia Medical Center, Fisherville and Charlottesville, Virginia
11. Thomas Jefferson University Medical Center and Magee Memorial Hospital, Philadelphia, Pennsylvania
12. New York University Medical Center, New York, New York
13. Boston University Medical Center, Boston, Massachusetts

Despite the number and location of these centers, they handle only about 15 percent of the new spinal injuries each year. Thus, the remainder of the persons with spinal injury in the United States receive care at the Veterans Administration Spinal Injury Centers or in community hospitals.

Veterans Administration Spinal Cord Injury Centers

Persons who have served in the United States military are eligible to receive care at a Veterans Administration hospital (VAH). Consequently, if a spinal injury is incurred during active service (service-connected disability), the disabled person will have a top priority for care at a VAH for the rest of his or her life and will receive a generous disability pension ($20,000 to $25,000 annually as of 1979) regardless of other income. A person who has veteran status and receives a spinal injury as a civilian (nonservice-connected disability) is also eligible for care at a VAH but receives a disability pension that decreases in amount as other income increases.

Spinal Injury Centers are part of VA hospitals in the following cities: Brockton, Massachusetts; Bronx, New York; Castle Point, New York; Cleveland, Ohio; East Orange, New Jersey; Hampton, Virginia; Hines, Illinois; Houston, Texas; Long Beach, California; Memphis, Tennessee; Miami, Florida; Palo Alto, California; Richmond, Virginia; San Juan, Puerto Rico; St. Louis, Missouri; Tampa, Florida; West Roxbury, Massachusetts; Wood, Wisconsin.

At these 18 spinal injury services, a total of 1,409 beds have been allocated for treatment of spinal injury. Many of the persons occupying those beds at any one time will have been readmitted for follow-up evaluation or for treatment of complications. Consequently, given an estimated 7,000 to 10,000 new spinal injuries nationally, a majority of these individuals will receive their acute management and rehabilitation in community hospitals.

Community Hospitals

Although estimates vary, it is probable that between 50 percent and 70 percent of the persons with new spinal injuries receive their acute management and rehabilitation training at a hospital in or near their own community. Experience indicates that persons with high cervical injuries have a higher probability of being referred to a regional spinal injury center and uncomplicated cases of quadriplegia and paraplegia are more likely to remain in the local area. Thus, whether or not a person is referred to a regional spinal injury center will depend on the level of the injury, the preferences of the primary care physician, and the wishes of the family. At this time, there is no evidence that treatment given at a regional spinal injury center is "better" than that given at a community hospital, but there is evidence that the total costs of the inpatient acute management and rehabilitation phase may be less at a regional spinal injury center than in the community. This cost differential is believed to relate to the prevention of medical complications and early mobilization of the person, the use of a systems approach to a complex syndrome such as spinal injury, and the specialized training of all members of the rehabilitation team.

WHO RECEIVES A SPINAL INJURY?

In conjunction with the development of the regional model spinal cord injury treatment system, the Rehabilitation Services Administration established the National Spinal Cord Injury Data Research Center in Phoenix, Arizona, in 1972. Data on all persons treated at the regional spinal injury centers are sent to Phoenix to become part of the common data base.

Based on the data collected from 1973 through 1977, some information about a large sample of the spinal injured population is becoming available (National Spinal Cord Injury Model Systems Conference 1978). However, since only 10 percent to 15 percent of the spinal injured population receives care through the regional system, and since those who do go through the regional system may not be a random sample of the spinal cord injury population, these data must be considered to be tentative.

Figure 1.2 presents striking information regarding age at injury. Almost 50 percent of the spinal injuries in this sample occurred between the ages of 15 and 24. Sixty-two percent occurred in the age range 15–29. Thus, the spinal cord injured group is predominantly a young one. Forty-eight percent of those reaching the regional spinal injury centers have paraplegia and 52 percent have quadriplegia (Young 1977). Whether this is a true ratio of paraplegia and quadriplegia in the population is not known at the present time. It should be recalled that there is reason to believe that persons with quadriplegia have a higher probability of being referred to a regional spinal injury center than persons with paraplegia.

The cause of injury for those who sustain a paraplegia and a quadriplegia is shown in table 1.1. Vehicular accident is the most frequent cause of spinal injury. It is interesting to note, however, the relative incidence of penetrating wounds and sports injuries as a cause of paraplegia and quadriplegia. One is more likely to receive a bullet or stab wound in the trunk and back region than in the neck region; thus, the incidence of paraplegia resulting from these events is much greater than quadriplegia. However, the incidence of quadriplegia as the result of a sports injury is over ten times greater than paraplegia. Diving, surfboarding, trampoline accidents, and skiing accidents are among those that produce quadriplegia.

Young (1977) has indicated that 82 percent of spinal injuries occur to males and 18 percent occur to females. Table 1.2 indicates that, for both sexes, vehicular accidents are the primary cause of spinal injury, although more females than males obtain their injury in this manner.

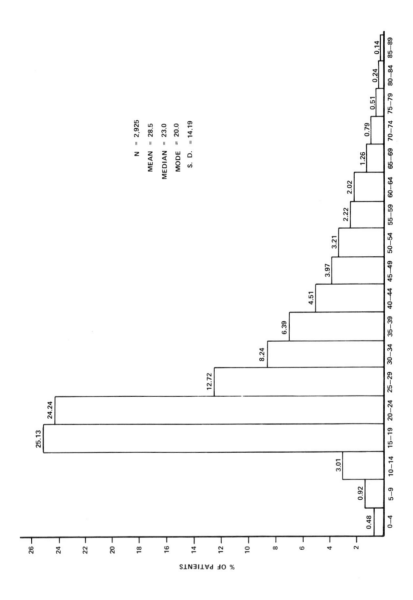

Fig. 1.2. Age at onset of spinal cord injury.
SOURCE: *National Spinal Cord Injury Model Systems Conference: Proceedings (1978)*.

Table 1.1. Incidence of Paraplegia and Quadriplegia by Cause of Injury

CAUSE OF INJURY	LEVEL OF SPINAL INJURY		
N = 2,821	Paraplegia	Quadriplegia	Both
Vehicular Accident	47.5%	46.5%	47.0%
Penetrating Wounds	20.9	6.3	13.3
Sports	2.3	26.4	14.8
Falls	24.9	17.3	21.0
Others	4.4	3.5	3.9
Total	100.0%	100.0%	100.0%

SOURCE: *National Spinal Cord Injury Model Systems Conference: Proceedings (1978).*

Table 1.2. Cause of Spinal Injury According to Sex

CAUSE OF INJURY	SEX OF THE SPINAL INJURED PERSON		
N = 2,854	Male	Female	Both
Vehicular Accidents	44.6%	57.4%	46.9%
Penetrating Wounds	13.0	14.4	13.2
Sports	16.3	8.4	14.9
Falls	22.4	14.6	21.0
Other	3.7	5.3	4.0
Total	100.0%	100.0%	100.0%

NOTE: Total incidence of males in national sample is 82 percent; females, 18 percent.
SOURCE: *National Spinal Cord Injury Model Systems Conference: Proceedings (1978).*

Cause of injury varies strikingly according to the ethnic or racial group of the individual, as revealed in table 1.3. Sports injuries account for a larger percentage of injuries within the white group than within other racial or ethnic groups, whereas penetrating wounds account for the greatest percentage of spinal injuries within the black group. The American Indian group obtains its spinal injuries from vehicular accidents almost exclusively. However, the overall representation of these ethnic or racial groups is unbalanced. Whites account for 77.3 percent of the sample; blacks, 13.8 percent; American Indians, 2.4 percent; Hispanics, 5.4 percent; and other groups, 1.1 percent (National Spinal Cord Injury Model Systems Conference 1978).

The cause of spinal injury varies with age, as revealed in table 1.4. For the age group 0-14, the causes of spinal injury are more evenly distributed than in other age groups. Vehicular accident accounts for the largest percentage of injuries within all age groups until age 60, at which point falls become the primary cause of spinal injury. In fact, falls account for an increasing percen-

Table 1.3. Cause of Injury for Different Racial and Ethnic Groups

CAUSE OF INJURY	RACE OR ETHNIC GROUP OF THE SPINAL INJURED PERSON					
N = 2,904	White	Black	Amer. Ind.	Hispanic	Other	All
Vehicular Accident	50.2%	27.0%	78.6%	37.3%	41.9%	46.9%
Penetrating Wounds	7.3	41.0	5.7	27.9	22.6	13.2
Sports	17.1	6.8	4.3	10.8	9.7	14.9
Falls	20.9	23.3	5.7	21.5	22.6	20.0
Other	4.5	2.0	5.7	2.5	3.2	4.1
Total	100.0%	100.0%	100.0%	100.0%	100.0%	100.0%

SOURCE: *National Spinal Cord Injury Model Systems Conference: Proceedings (1978).*

Table 1.4. Cause of Spinal Injury within Different Age Groups

CAUSE OF INJURY	AGE CATEGORY					
N = 2,904	0-14	15-29	30-44	45-59	60-74	75-89
Vehicular Accident	29.7%	50.8%	42.2%	43.1%	41.0%	30.8%
Penetrating Wounds	28.1	12.6	16.8	8.4	2.6	—
Sports	23.4	19.3	9.2	1.5	—	—
Falls	16.4	14.2	27.0	40.1	48.7	50.0
Other	2.4	3.1	4.9	7.0	7.7	19.2
Total	100.0%	100.0%	100.0%	100.0%	100.0%	100.0%

SOURCE: *National Spinal Cord Injury Model Systems Conference: Proceedings (1978).*

tage of spinal injuries after age 30, whereas sports injuries decline as a factor in spinal injury as age increases.

The National Spinal Cord Injury Model Systems Conference (1978) revealed other interesting facts about this sample of persons with spinal injury. Fifty-three percent of these persons are single at onset of spinal injury and 33 percent are married. Divorce, separation, and widowhood account for 14 percent. The educational attainments at onset of injury include:

8th Grade or Less	16.3%
Some High School	28.4%
Completed High School or Equivalent Diploma	34.2%
Some College	14.1%
Bachelor's Degree	4.3%
Postgraduate Work	2.7%

Thus, 55.3 percent of these persons with spinal injury have a high school education or more at the time of their injury. Furthermore, at time of injury, 58.1 percent of the sample were working and 23.4 percent held a student status.

Consequently, it appears that the group of persons with spinal injury are predominantly male, quite young and active, with a history of productive educational and vocational endeavors. As a group they tend to be fairly well educated by the time that they receive their spinal injuries. Twenty percent of the group is female; they are also young and fairly well educated.

However, these active and dynamic people who are often in the midst of mapping out a career or course of action that will characterize their adult life suddenly find themselves paralyzed, with no feeling in their limbs, and with no control over their bladder or bowel. Life as he or she had known it will be interrupted by months of hospitalization and an often lengthy period during which new techniques must be mastered as a necessity for survival and independent function. The person must learn how to deal with a world de-signed for and dominated by able-bodied persons who are not very accepting of those with disabilities. He must learn to face people who now communicate that he is different than he used to be and perhaps ''less'' than he used to be. He must learn new types of recreation and leisure time activities and, perhaps, a new vocation. However following an educational or vocational training pro-gram, he must learn to face potential employers who do not want to hire him, not because he is not qualified but because he is disabled. He must learn that many of his previous friends drift away from him and he must seek opportunities to meet new people and make new friends. Yet strangers tend to avoid any interaction with him; thus, he must learn techniques to put others at ease and he must teach them to forget that he is in a wheelchair. He must learn to retain some sense of humor in order to cope with the daily frustrations and hard work that living with a disability entails. And he must learn to maintain some sense of dignity and self-worth when faced with a social welfare system that penalizes efforts to become independent and self-sufficient. These, then, are some of the issues that constitute the impact of a disability.

2
Rehabilitation as a Behavior Change Process

A major premise of this book is that *rehabilitation is the process of learning to live with one's disability in one's own environment*. This learning experience is a dynamic process that starts at the moment of injury and continues for the remainder of the person's life. There is no definable end point that can be labeled as "rehabilitated" or "adjusted" because, as with all people in all areas of life, disabled persons are continually learning to adapt to their environment in, hopefully, more functional and satisfying ways. And it may take many years to incorporate all of the changes that spinal injury brings into one's life. Carter (1977) believes that the newly injured person requires at least 18 to 20 months before the new ADL and mobility techniques become a fairly automatic part of the person's daily routine. At this point, the person is ready to begin the challenges of an educational or vocational program.

Learning to live with a disability appears to be a lengthy and often frustrating process. No matter how long a person has been injured, he or she never ceases to get irritated, frustrated, and perhaps depressed over the inconveniences that the disability entails—e.g., finding one's clothing is wet with urine when one is hurrying to get to an appointment on time (Consumer Conference 1977). However, in order to continue to face these repeated frustrations, there have to be some rewards and satisfactions in life. Everyone needs a reason to get out of bed in the morning; there have to be some fulfillments in the life of a disabled person for him or her to continue to endure the fatigue and frustration that life with a physical disability may include. Consequently, we must examine the rehabilitation process to determine how successful we have been at helping people to achieve some degree of happiness in their lives.

SUICIDE AND SELF-NEGLECT

Data from several follow-up studies suggest that not everyone does find sufficient rewards in life after the onset of a spinal cord injury. Some persons commit suicide and some cease to care for their bodies and commit "physiological suicide" through self-neglect (Seymour 1955).

Wilcox and Stauffer (1972) followed 423 consecutive patients with spinal injury admitted to Rancho Los Amigos Hospital from January 1 through December 31, 1967. In this sample, there were 50 deaths; 17 (34 percent) occurred from avoidable conditions, such as overdose of drugs and/or alcohol, suicide, and multiple pressure sores with severe infections. Ninety-four percent of these deaths occurred before the sixth anniversary of the injury. No patient in this group was married at the time of death. Forty-seven percent of this group had some history of the use of drugs. No data on the incidence of paraplegia or quadriplegia among these deaths are given.

Nyquist and Bors (1967) report a follow-up study of United States veterans with traumatic spinal cord injury during the period 1946–1965. They note that provable suicide occurred in 8.1 percent of the 258 deaths. Forty-three percent of these suicides occurred within five years of the date of injury. They state that two of the deaths that were labeled as accidental might have been suicide, and seven deaths were associated with alcohol or drug abuse. Combining these figures with the known suicides suggests that as many as 12 percent of the deaths may have resulted from the person's own actions. Because of the manner in which they report the data, it is impossible to determine what percentage of the deaths from other physiological causes may have been hastened by self-neglect. Thus, the data from Nyquist and Bors should be considered to be a conservative estimate of the mortality rate in spinal cord injury in which behavioral factors played a role.

Hopkins (1971) found that the suicide rate for the disabled was higher than for the general population, but her hypothesis that the suicide rate would increase as severity of disability increased was not supported. However, her conclusions must be considered to be tentative, and this issue requires further study. To reach her conclusion, she compared suicide data of amputees among Finnish war veterans during the 20-year period, 1945–1965, with the Nyquist and Bors (1967) data on spinal cord injury during the same period and found a higher suicide rate among the Finnish amputees. However, such cross-cultural comparisons must be interpreted with extreme caution because of the number of unknown and uncontrolled variables involved. For example, the base rate of suicide in the Finnish versus American culture may be different, and the postwar economic circumstances in the two countries may have been quite different. Nevertheless, Hopkins has made an important contribution to the field by writing one of the only papers exploring the topic of suicide in the population of persons with spinal cord injury.

Kerr and Thompson (1972) present data on the death rate among individuals with spinal cord injury whose mental adjustment was rated as bad, poor, or fair. The cause of death was not reported nor were the criteria for rating mental adjustment. However, it is striking to note that 74 percent of the deaths in their follow-up sample occurred in persons who had not been successful in "adjusting'' to the disability. Of the deaths among those not adjusting to the spinal injury, 80 percent occurred in persons beyond the age of 45. It is not clear in their report, but apparently this refers to age at follow-up rather than age at injury. No information on duration or severity of disability is presented.

Price (1973) analyzed the causes of 11 deaths in a sample of 227 persons with spinal cord injury and found that psychological factors contributed to the death in over half of the cases. She concludes:

> The primary concern for patients with spinal cord injury had traditionally been focussed upon physical and vocational rehabilitation. The importance of these facets of rehabilitation is undeniable. However, the influence of emotional disability upon the cause of death in six of eleven patients, emphasizes the need for better use of available methods of prediction and the development of new tools for coping with the emotional needs of the severely handicapped. (Price 1973, p. 220)

It would appear, according to these studies, that between 12 percent and 50 percent of deaths among persons with spinal injury may be related to self-destructive behavior. However, we need follow-up data that identify more carefully the characteristics of those who have hastened their own deaths. From these studies, it would appear that the first five years following injury are critical ones in which the person needs tremendous assistance in reentering the adult world, this time as a disabled person. Older individuals and those who are not married may need particular attention from professionals, both because the task of adjustment may seem overwhelming when one is older and when one is alone. Relevant issues to be studied include: duration of disability, severity of disability, preinjury adjustment history, age, marital status, and all the other variables that might help us to understand this group. For example, financial security may be an important issue.

Any study of United States veterans must be interpreted with some caution since a certain percentage of the sample may have much greater financial security than a civilian sample of persons with spinal cord injury. Many veterans with a service-connected spinal injury may receive at least $20,000 a year as of 1979. Thus, it is interesting to note that Nyquist and Bors (1967) reported the lowest suicide rate of the above studies.

In addition to suicide, the death rate in persons who seem to have trouble living with the disability is a major concern. Kerr and Thompson (1972) and Price (1973) both report the influence of psychological factors in a large proportion of the deaths in their studies. Hallin (1968) at the Kenney Rehabilitation Institute states:

> In conducting a follow-up clinic for patients with spinal cord injuries who had been discharged after going through the rehabilitation process, we have become persuaded that psychological adjustment, rather than intellectual capacity or the level or completeness of injury, is the critical factor in determining rehabilitation success. Once a patient has been discharged, his fluid intake, his bowel and bladder needs, and the health of his skin are his responsibility, and he will accept this responsibility only if he accepts his disabled body and values himself and his remaining function enough to avoid preventable complications. Without this acceptance, the most intensive therapy programme and the most ideal voca-

tional plan will be of little overall benefit to him. With it, he not only can avoid regressing but can proceed with education, work, or whatever avenues of living are open to him. (Hallin 1968, p. 128)

Given these data and opinions, we must examine the rehabilitation process to seek ways to improve the delivery of services to persons with spinal injury. Despite our good intentions, it would appear that we are not completely successful at teaching people to live with their disabilities in their own environments in such a way that they can have the opportunity to find rewards and satisfactions in their lives. Perhaps our task must be not only to teach ADL and mobility techniques, but to teach a person to find a reason for getting out of bed in the morning. Although we cannot give a person a reason to continue to live, perhaps we can teach the person how to go about finding one for himself.

Traditionally, the focus of rehabilitation has been on ADL and mobility techniques, but bathing, grooming, toileting, eating, and getting about physically are the skills that an average five-year-old has mastered in our culture. Successful adult functioning requires more than ADL and mobility skills; it requires the ability to interact socially in quite sophisticated ways, to compete successfully with one's peers in social, recreational, educational, vocational, and economic spheres. Thus, it would appear that the content of the traditional rehabilitation program has been inadequate to meet the needs of disabled persons. Furthermore, it is proposed that this very delimited focus of rehabilitation derives from the use of the medical model of rehabilitation rather than the learning model.

MODELS OF REHABILITATION SERVICE DELIVERY

Within the field of health care delivery, the medical model has been the predominant approach for most of the history of modern medicine. However, recently there has been growing concern that the medical model may be the approach of choice for certain disease categories but that the learning model is much more appropriate for teaching health care behaviors (Goffman 1961; Friedson 1970; Carlson 1975; Howard and Strauss 1975; Lapatra 1975; Illich 1976). The consensus is that "health is a condition for which the individual must take prime responsibility himself" (Rushmer 1975, p. 177). Furthermore, in the field of rehabilitation, Anderson (1978) has proposed that the educational frame of reference has been overshadowed by the medical-surgical approach, yet it is the training aspect that makes rehabilitation unique. Thus, let us examine the rehabilitation process and evaluate the utility of these two models as strategies of effective service delivery.

In the first several weeks after the onset of spinal cord injury, survival of the patient is the concern of the hospital personnel, and the person becomes the passive recipient of treatments designed to fix his body, i.e., skeletal traction or surgery for the spinal injury, treatment of associated injuries, procedures to prevent skin problems, management of bladder and bowel functions, and respiratory assists if breathing is a problem. When medical stability has been achieved, when the person is no longer sick but only physically disabled, a rehabilitation program is outlined that will teach the person how to manage the activities of daily living and the mobility techniques needed to get around in the world. Bed mobility, transfers in and out of the wheelchair, use of the wheelchair, possibly ambulation and driving a car with hand controls are the usual mobility techniques taught. At this point, the person can no longer be the passive recipient of treatments dispensed but must become an active participant in the process of learning to live with the spinal injury.

However, hospitals are designed to dispense units of organic treatment (Trieschmann 1975). During acute illnesses, the person can be a passive recipient of care and, when recovered, leave the hospital and resume his life with no ill effects of the treatment approach. But with spinal cord injury, any system that focuses on dispensing units of treatment may implicitly treat the person as the passive recipient of treatment, and this may conflict with the active participation that we say is so important. If one considers the type of statistics that various departments in rehabilitation centers keep for accountability purposes, the emphasis on units of treatment becomes apparent: number of beds filled, number of days of hospitalization, number of patients seen in therapy each day, number of hot packs applied, number of patients seen for ADL training, number of treatments given, number of electromyographic studies performed, number of placements made, number of group therapy sessions held, number of patients seen for counseling, number of intermittent catheterizations performed, number of hand splints made.

If performance of the various rehabilitation departments is measured in such terms, this may suggest that we believe that the giving of treatments, the dispensing of units of care, will lead to the improved ability of the person with spinal injury to manage life outside of the hospital. This, then, is the essence of the medical model. If we implicitly treat the person as the passive recipient of units of therapy in the rehabilitation hospital, how can we expect the person to be an active participant in life outside of the hospital?

In the medical model, the behavioral equation for rehabilitation success consists of:

$$B = f (O \times p)$$

Behavior is a function of treatments to the organic variables (O) unless hindered by underlying personality problems (p). As presented in figure 2.1, units of treatment are given to the organic variables (O), such as the skin, bladder and bowel, paralysis, lack of sensation, respiratory function, etc. The (p) is defined as lack of motivation, depression, low self-esteem, low self-confidence, anxiety, anger, frustration, dependency. Units of treatment

$B= f (O \times p)$

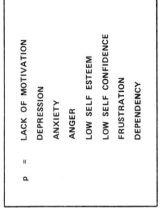

p = LACK OF MOTIVATION

DEPRESSION

ANXIETY

ANGER

LOW SELF ESTEEM

LOW SELF CONFIDENCE

FRUSTRATION

DEPENDENCY

UNITS OF TREATMENT

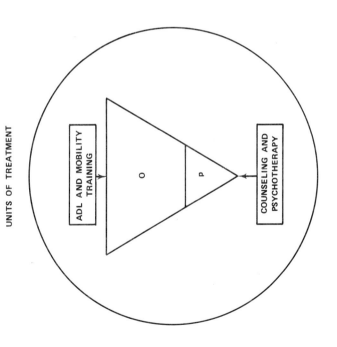

ADL AND MOBILITY TRAINING

O

p

COUNSELING AND PSYCHOTHERAPY

are delivered to the (p) variables also in the form of counseling and psychotherapy. The major (p) variable of concern is that of motivation, often synonymous with cooperation. The person may be labeled as unmotivated if he is too much the passive recipient of treatments or if he expects to be too much of an active participant in the decisions about his program.

There is great variability in the extent to which individual rehabilitation personnel and rehabilitation departments expect the person to be a passive recipient of treatment, but it is sufficiently prevalent to warrant attention. Persons with spinal injury have cited repeated examples of their exclusion from the decision-making process regarding their care and future, their inability to receive information about their physical status or about the program planned for them, and the unwillingness of many rehabilitation personnel to listen to their ideas about how a task could be accomplished more efficiently. In addition, they have been frustrated by the double message given to them by rehabilitation centers: you must learn to take care of your body but all decisions will be made for you (Consumer Conference 1977). In substantiation of this observation, Rushmer states that, ''Most physicians seem to share the unstated assumption that patients are more easily managed if they are kept in an optimal state of ignorance'' (Rushmer 1975, p. 179).

In contrast to the medical model is the educational model of rehabilitation, the learning approach. Within this approach, rehabilitation is viewed as the *process* of *teaching* the person to live with his disability in his *own environment*. It is a learning process and everyone on the rehabilitation staff functions as a teacher. The focus of all of our rehabilitation efforts is the behavior of the person with spinal injury, and his behavior is the only outcome by which the success and failure of our efforts can be judged. The person must be an active participant in this process, and a rehabilitation program must be designed by the staff *with*, not for, the person to meet his needs in terms of who he is and from what environment he comes and to which he will return.

If rehabilitation is the process of teaching the person to live with his disability in his own environment, then the principles of learning and the multiple factors that influence behavior become the concern of everyone on the rehabilitation team. Within this approach, performance of the rehabilitation departments must be measured in terms of functional gains in the behavior of the person, regardless of the number of treatments administered. Thus, a behavioral contract may be the logical solution.

In the learning model, figure 2.2, the behavioral equation for rehabilitation success is:

$$B = f (P \times O \times E)$$

Behavior is a function of the person, the organism, and the environment. Figure 2.3 displays some of the variables influencing the behavior of the person with spinal cord injury, the person variables, the organismic variables,

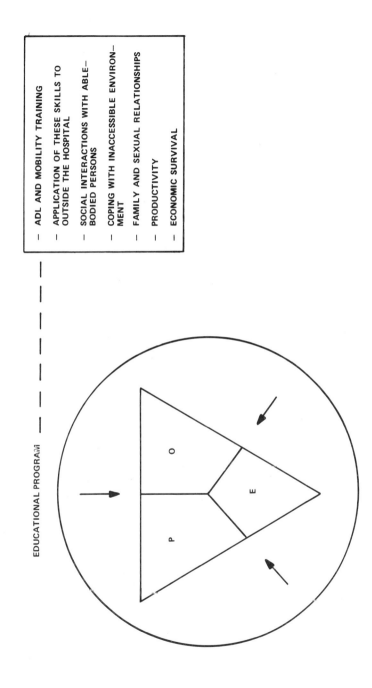

B = f (P × O × E)

EDUCATIONAL PROGRAM

- ADL AND MOBILITY TRAINING
- APPLICATION OF THESE SKILLS TO OUTSIDE THE HOSPITAL
- SOCIAL INTERACTIONS WITH ABLE-BODIED PERSONS
- COPING WITH INACCESSIBLE ENVIRON-MENT
- FAMILY AND SEXUAL RELATIONSHIPS
- PRODUCTIVITY
- ECONOMIC SURVIVAL

Fig. 2.2. The learning model (P = person; O = organism; E = environment).

27

P = Person Variables

Repertoire of habits
Personality style
Types of rewards
Internal vs. external locus of control
Method of coping with stress
Self-image
Creativity

O = Organic Variables

Age
Severity of disability
Medical complications
Congenital anomalies
Strength
Endurance

E = Environmental Variables

Hospital milieu
Stigma value of disability
Family and interpersonal support
Financial security
Social milieu
Urban vs. rural residence
Access to medical attention and equipment repair
Access to educational, recreational, and avocational pursuits
Socioeconomic status
Architectural barriers and availability of transportation
Legislation
Cultural and ethnic influences

Fig. 2.3. $B = f (P \times O \times E)$. Behavior is a function of the Person (**P**), the Organism (**O**), and the Environment (**E**).

and the environmental variables. For purposes of this discussion, the organic variables are assumed to be constant. Therefore, using this educational model, the learning model, the emphasis is on the $P \times E$, the Person-Environment interaction, as the key to producing behavior change.

Although the topic of motivation will be discussed in the next chapter, it is important to note that the management of motivational deficits varies in these two models. Within the medical model, when motivation is lacking, it is defined as a problem that the psychologist is asked to solve in his or her office. The traditional unit of treatment given is psychotherapy or counseling, but these treatments have been unsuccessful at improving motivational level (Diamond, Weiss, and Grynbaum 1968). But in the learning model, motivation is less of a problem because it is treated by modifying the $P \times E$, Person-Environment interaction (Fordyce 1971; Margolin 1971; Trieschmann 1975, 1976, 1978b; Willems 1976a). In addition, by placing our emphasis on the $P \times E$, Person-Environment interaction, we have a methodology for teaching the person to find some rewards in life to offset the daily frustrations that disability entails.

Furthermore, within the medical model, if the person does not seem to participate at the level at which he is judged to be capable, he is labeled unmotivated. It is the patient's failure; he lacks the inner drive to get better.

However, within the learning model, if the person does not seem to participate at the level at which he is judged to be capable, it is the program that is the problem. Obviously, the proper rewards are not available for which the person will work. In the former case, the patient is the failure; in the latter case, the program is a failure.

Historically, the medical model has derived from the disease or sickness orientation within the practice of medicine. There is an underlying pathology that will be remedied through units of treatment. In the management of the acute spinal injury, the medical model may be appropriate. The spinal cord has been damaged and various units of treatment are administered to prevent further damage, to assist the vertebral column in healing, to maintain adequate drainage of urine from the bladder, to prevent pressure sores, and to maintain proper respiration. However, when the vertebral column has healed and other associated injuries have healed, the individual is no longer "sick." He is a healthy person who happens to have some paralyzed muscles, lack of sensation, and impaired control over bladder and bowel. There is no further treatment that can be administered to heal these dysfunctions. Therefore, the rehabilitation phase begins. However, the content and focus of the program will be quite different depending on which model of rehabilitation is used.

In the medical model of rehabilitation, the content and focus will still be one of remedying some underlying pathology. As exhibited in figure 2.1, units of treatment will be directed at both (O) variables and (p) variables. The content will be ADL and mobility training almost exclusively since the assumption is made that with these skills the person will be equipped to cope with the world outside of the hospital. If the person displays anxiety, self-doubt, depression, temper outbursts, lack of motivation, the medical model is again applied. A personality problem has been identified; the remedy is psychotherapy or counseling. The implicit assumption is made that these behaviors are evidence of some pathology rather than a very realistic reaction to a sudden disability.

However, in the learning model, it is assumed that the person is healthy but now must learn a series of behaviors so that he or she can return to the world outside of the hospital. Thus, the initial step is a very thorough evaluation of who the person is, what the impact of the disability is on this unique individual, and to what environment will he or she return. What are the environmental resources? What needs to be learned in order to achieve some success in life and some rewards from life? As exhibited in figure 2.2, an educational program will be designed to help the person compete in a world designed for and dominated by able-bodied people. ADL and mobility training will be part of the program but only one small part. They are not ends in themselves but rather are means to an end. Therefore, the application of ADL and mobility skills to survival in the world outside of the hospital, social skills training, training in maintaining family and sexual relationships, a focus on the multiple dimensions of productivity, and economic survival will be the content of the rehabilitation program.

Berk and Feibel (1978) did a follow-up study of 85 disabled persons who had been discharged from a rehabilitation center six months previously. Thirty-seven percent reported serious depression and 32 percent reported significant anxiety. In terms of life outside of the hospital, 43 percent reported a decrease in time spent in community activities and 56 percent experienced a decrease in or complete absence of socialization with family and friends. However, 50 percent reported that they had received little or no help in working out their social, financial, and emotional problems, whereas only 13 percent were dissatisfied with the amount of help they had received with ADL skills. Families were affected as well; 52 percent of the families reported that normal family functioning had been disrupted by the disability and that this was resented. Yet, families also reported that they had not received enough help with adjustment issues relative to the disability, although they thought that the ADL training had been satisfactory.

In a similar vein, Udin and Keith (1978) followed a group of 60 disabled persons who were discharged into their homes and noted the content and frequency of various daily activities. Their results showed that most daily activities were restricted to in and around the home, interpersonal contacts were restricted to family members, and the person's behavior was predominantly self-oriented and passive. Most expressed great frustration or depression about the passive and unfulfilling quality of their daily routine.

> If the objective of rehabilitation, to encourage as normal a life style as possible, is to be met, more emphasis must be put on skills in the constructive use of leisure time and social interaction. These skills are predominantly developed in recreation, psychological, and social service therapies, not in the functionally oriented physical and occupational therapies which are given the greatest priority during an inpatient program. All services should place more emphasis, as well, on functioning in home and community settings. It is clearly there that we must look for the results of rehabilitation and to learn about potential alternatives to current programs. (Udin and Keith 1978, pp. 19-20)

A MULTIVARIATE APPROACH TO THE CONCEPT OF ADJUSTMENT

The purpose of this book is to describe a model of rehabilitation that will assist persons with the process of achieving maximal function and satisfaction in life outside of the hospital and to discuss the multitude of variables that will ultimately influence this process. In the remainder of this book, these variables will be identified, the results of research will be evaluated, and the observations and judgments of persons with spinal injury will be offered in an attempt to determine what we know and particularly what we do not know about the process of adjustment to spinal injury. These variables will be artificially separated into separate chapters, but any one behavior under discussion will also be influenced by other variables. Furthermore, it is difficult to understand a behavior without considering the environment in which it occurs. Consequently, the person-environment interaction will be a key focus of the discussion.

Much of the research that will be presented constitutes examples of cross-sectional research rather than longitudinal research. Thus, the results of behavior on one occasion must be generalized to the multitude of sequentially spaced episodes that are involved in the process of living with a disability, and the potential for error may be great. Consequently, an underlying theme of this book is that,

> The patient's behavior is like a continuous stream that sometimes damps down to a minimal level and sometimes quickens to a very brisk pace, sometimes widens or even splits into several simultaneous occurrences and sometimes narrows to one, sometimes intertwines with the behavior of others, and sometimes moves in isolation, sometimes changes form or direction at the patient's initiative and sometimes at the instigation of others. Each of the discrete events in that stream occurs at some unique place and time, and yet the stream as a whole flows in a continuous sequential manner over time. (Willems 1976a, p. 216)

Part II
Adjustment to Spinal Cord Injury: The State of the Art

3

Psychological Factors in the Adjustment to Spinal Cord Injury

One of the objectives of this book is to identify what is known and what is not known about the process of adjustment to spinal cord injury. However, it is difficult to be definitive concerning what is known about the process of adjustment because of the variation in the quality of the research that has been conducted to date. An unfortunate number of studies have methodological flaws that make interpretation of the results tentative at best. Thus, many of the results reported below can only be considered to represent hypotheses that require further testing.

FLAWS IN RESEARCH DESIGN

A detailed discussion of problems of research design and methodology will be presented in chapter 10. However, some key problems must be mentioned here since they may complicate the interpretation of the results in any one study. This is not an exhaustive listing of flaws in research but merely a summary of the major problems.

Subjects

An unfortunate number of studies assume that the population of persons with spinal cord injury is a homogeneous one. However, there is sufficient evidence to suggest that this is not the case and that there is greater heterogeneity than may have been believed. Therefore, until the critical subject variables have been identified, the sample of subjects should be described in great detail.

Some of the subject variables that should be considered are:

1. *Age*. Average age is often reported, whereas it is known that age of onset of spinal injury forms a skewed distribution (National Spinal Cord Injury Model Systems Conference 1978). More spinal injuries occur in the age group 15-19 than any other, but there are enough cases in the older age groups to warrant separate study.

2. *Duration of Disability*. This variable is not always reported. Yet can it be assumed that there is no difference in the behavior of a person injured for one year versus a person injured for six years?

3. *Sex*. Spinal cord injury occurs to males four times more frequently than to females; thus, in any one study there will be very few females available. However, until it is known whether sex differences are important to the adjustment process, this variable should be specified.

4. *Socioeconomic Status*. There is some evidence that this variable may be a significant factor in reaction to disability; therefore, it should be specified in descriptions of subject populations.

5. *Severity of Disability*. Since it is not known if paraplegia and quadriplegia are similar in the types of adjustments required, it is not appropriate to combine the groups into one sample without analyzing the data for differences according to level of injury.

6. *Etiology of the Disability*. Some studies combine traumatic and nontraumatic spinal cord injuries, including poliomyelitis and multiple sclerosis, into one sample of subjects and attempt to describe the psychological adjustment of this heterogeneous group. Because of a similarity of physical symptoms (spinal cord dysfunction), a similarity in psychological adjustment processes is assumed. This assumption is not warranted.

7. *Financial Security*. Financial security may influence the process of adjustment to spinal cord injury. Therefore, any study on United States veterans should include data on the number of disabilities that are service-connected and non-service-connected. The difference in the financial security of these two groups will be great. In addition, because of this factor it is difficult to generalize the results of studies on veterans to the civilian population who do not have similar financial benefits.

Methodology

When one reads some of the publications on the adjustment to spinal cord injury, one has to assume that some of the researchers never took a course in basic experimental design or, if they did, they have forgotten what they learned. Thus, the following is a summary of some of the methodological flaws in the research that make interpretation of the results difficult:

1. *Control Groups*. Some studies should have control groups but they do not.

2. *Base Rates*. Base rates are the average frequency of occurrence of a

characteristic in the population. Inattention to base rates may result in the erroneous attribution of a characteristic to persons with quadriplegia or paraplegia, though the incidence of the characteristic is no greater in spinal cord injury than in other groups.

3. *Test Instruments and Rating Scales.* Some researchers devise a rating scale for measuring the criterion variable but present no data on validity of the instrument. These studies presume that reliability insures validity, although an unfortunate number do not provide data on reliability either.

4. *Judges Who Rate the Criterion Variable.* Some studies use various rehabilitation personnel as judges to rate the presence or absence of the criterion variable (frequently defined as "adjustment" or depression). Yet evidence suggests that rehabilitation personnel are not accurate at rating psychological processes and consistently tend to overestimate the degree of psychological distress present.

5. *Criterion Variable.* Some studies use "adjustment to disability" as the criterion variable, and it is often measured by judges' ratings. However, the behaviors that should be used to assess "adjustment" are not specified; thus, patients may be rated by different judges on different behaviors. Furthermore, adjustment to disability is sometimes rated while the person is still hospitalized, which implicitly equates adjustment to disability with cooperation with hospital procedures.

6. *Interpretation of Nonsignificant Statistics.* An unfortunate number of researchers interpret results even though they failed to reach statistical significance. The researcher always justifies this procedure by stating that the data are in the direction predicted by the hypothesis, which only makes the error more egregious.

Investigator Paradigm Effect

Barber (1976) points out that most researchers are influenced by a paradigm when they plan a research project. A paradigm is defined as a body of assumptions, beliefs, and related methods and techniques that are shared by a group of scientists at any one time. Psychoanalytic theory and Skinnerian operant conditioning would be two examples of paradigms in psychology. The assumptions of the paradigm govern the choice of problems to be studied and define the "correct" methods for evaluating the problem. It defines what questions are asked and the means of obtaining an answer. Barber believes that the investigator paradigm effect plays a role in the planning and implementation of all research. Thus, in the research to be reported, any paradigm that seems to have acted as a "blinder" to alternative interpretations of the obtained data will be identified.

Many of these problems in research design are present in varying degrees in some of the studies reviewed throughout this book. The occurrence of these problems will be noted as the study is reviewed if their presence complicates the interpretation of the results. The intent is not to criticize any researcher personally but rather to indicate the improvements in research methodology that will be necessary if the state of the art is to be advanced.

EMOTIONAL REACTIONS AT ONSET
OF SPINAL CORD INJURY

Our knowledge of the immediate psychological consequences of spinal cord injury is incomplete. Wittkower, Gingras, Mergler, Wigdor, and Lepine (1954) compare the immediate reactions of soldiers and civilians to injury. Those injured during combat may show a certain amount of equanimity about the injury since they may be very glad just to be alive, and, second, the injury signifies the end of the war to them. Wittkower and associates state that whether the injury was sustained by action in a war or through accident, most persons with paraplegia feel, upon receiving the injury, that their legs have been cut off. However, seeing their legs and being able to touch them rekindles the hope that everything will be all right. ''Denial has begun to play its role; it is usually intense, and a major defense mechanism. This involuntary denial is so intense that, even after neurosurgical exploration reveals a hopelessly damaged cord, hope still remains'' (Wittkower et al. 1954, pp. 110-11).

Unfortunately, Wittkower and associates have equated the defense mechanism of denial with hope. This assumption is not necessary and represents an overinterpretation of the data, the data in this study appearing to be the descriptive impressions of the authors based on their ''knowledge'' of 50 cases of spinal cord lesions. Although their observations should be interpreted with caution, the concept of the differential implications of an injury sustained during combat versus civilian life is very interesting. Whether or not this factor has any long-term implications for adjustment to the disability in veterans remains to be determined. However, the person injured during combat does receive a pension that will provide financial security for life.

Heilporn and Noel (1968) reported that 53 percent of the 40 cases of traumatic spinal cord injury studied by them were conscious of the paralysis at the time of the accident. In 58 percent of the cases, disturbances of sensation were noticed after they became aware of the motor disability. Five percent (2 cases) perceived the anesthesia before noticing the motor paralysis. Thirteen percent reported apparent disturbances of the body image. Twenty percent had temporary pains for an undefined period of time following injury. The authors concluded that body image is not spontaneously modified after disconnection of the sensory path. The implications of their data for rehabilitation and psychological adjustment were deferred by the authors pending further study. They did not give any information about the sample other than the number of cases. Information was collected by interview and the interval between interview and onset of the disability is unspecified.

There are many individuals with spinal cord injury who report that they were immediately aware that they could not move following their accident. Valens' (1966) book about Jill Kinmont, the skier, describes her awareness of the paralysis, along with her inability to feel the coldness of the snow after her fall. Israel Goldiamond (1973) notes that he was aware of his inability to move as he lay on the ground beside his damaged automobile. Both persons reported what might be interpreted as temporary body image distortion. Jill Kinmont reports feeling armless until she had a good look at her arms in the operating room at the hospital. After a complete visualization of her arms, the armless feeling never recurred (Valens 1966).

While some percentage of persons who suffer a spinal cord injury are aware of their inability to move at the time of the accident, some are not aware. What percentages fall into each category we do not know definitely, but Heilporn and Noel's (1968) sample suggests that 50 percent could fall into each category. Why 50 percent of the injury cases were not aware of the paralysis has not yet been studied. In what percentage of these cases is the person unconscious for physical reasons and in what percentage of the cases did the person actively shut out the awareness of his inability to move? In studies into this issue, it will be important to differentiate between no report of awareness of motor paralysis upon question at time of injury or soon after versus not remembering an awareness of the paralysis when questioned weeks, months, or years later. It would be interesting to correlate early versus late ''awareness'' of paralysis with the process of adjusting to the spinal cord injury. Does an early awareness of the paralysis (regardless of how much hope of recovery is present) portend a ''better'' or ''easier'' adjustment to the disability? We do not know.

It would appear that in most cases of spinal cord injury, the initial awareness of the accident and its concomitants is superseded by a period (of varying duration) in which the person is not that alert or aware of what is going on about him. Is this a psychological state of shock which represents an ''unconscious protection against too massive or too rapid a perception of the traumatic and overwhelming reality'' as described by Gunther (1969, p. 98)? Or is this state a somewhat natural response caused by anesthesia for surgery and various medications for pain and other problems, in addition to the physical shock to the organism after experiencing an insult of sufficient magnitude to damage the spinal cord? Or is it a result of both psychological and physical factors? We do not know. However, the predominant emphasis in the literature is to give a psychological interpretation to this stage (Nagler 1950; Gunther 1969; Siller 1969; Knorr and Bull 1970; Kerr and Thompson 1972) if it is discussed at all.

Harris, Patel, Greer, and Naughton (1973) provide an excellent description of the psychological reactions to acute spinal paralysis which highlights some of the physical parameters influencing the newly injured person's behavior: ''Pain is very often the main problem and in our experience very often outweighs all other considerations in the patient's mind at this time, as he or she wonders if pain will be present for the rest of their life'' (Harris et al. 1973,

p. 132). They state that approximately 30 percent of patients with serious traumatic spinal injury have significant associated injury, usually a head injury. As a result the person may be unconscious initially, followed by a period of amnesia and confusion. In high cervical injury or with an associated chest injury, use of a respirator or performance of a tracheostomy can be very frightening, and the primary concern of these patients and their families is survival. Proper management of the acute injury may require geographical separation from family and loved ones (frightening situation) in order to get specialized care. Thus Harris and his associates recommended making arrangements for the family to have overnight accommodations at the hospital. Complete immobilization of the patient provides an ideal situation for the sensory deprivation syndrome and this should be prevented since it is very distressing to the patient and the staff.

Sensory deprivation as a possible factor in the person's behavior during the early stages of hospitalization has also been mentioned by Symington and Fordyce (1965), Das (1969), and McDaniel (1976). Symington and Fordyce refer to the profoundly altered sensory inputs from the lower part of the body. Alteration of sensory inputs and an absence of a significant proportion of sensory inputs occurs, both of which could be psychologically disruptive.

Das (1969) describes the feelings of panic that a person with quadriplegia can experience when faced with an abrupt loss of sensation over a majority of his body. He states that counseling by persons who have adjusted to their quadriplegia does not necessarily remove the feelings of panic. Thus, Das recommends an increase in stimulation over those areas of the body in which sensation remains and increases in stimulation of other sensory modalities, auditory and visual. McDaniel (1976) emphasizes the need to consider sensory isolation, restriction of movement, and sensory deprivation as key determinants of the behavior of ill and physically disabled persons during long hospitalization.

Since data on sensory deprivation in persons with spinal injury are not available currently, research into this process in nondisabled college students may provide some clues as to which areas should be studied in persons with disabilities. Zubek (1969) has amassed a great deal of data on sensory deprivation, and this book should be useful to any researcher or clinician who works with persons with spinal injury.

Although Zubeck (1969) cautions that many of the studies cited provide sometimes conflicting results because of differences in the experimental methodology, some of these results might provide hypotheses for research into the immediate reaction to spinal cord injury.

1. Restriction of movement does produce some stress, particularly bodily discomforts and thinking difficulties, but sensory deprivation in addition to restriction of movement is associated with significantly more stress.

2. Physical exercise during perceptual deprivation is associated with

significantly less impairment on intellectual and perceptual motor tests and fewer EEG changes in contrast to no exercise at all.

3. Two weeks of perceptual deprivation is associated with a progressive decrease in mean occipital lobe frequencies on the EEG. The EEG frequencies begin to increase when perceptual stimulation increases, but even after ten days, they may remain below normal level. Correlated with the magnitude of the EEG changes are motivational losses, such as an inability to study or engage in purposeful activity.

4. There is a great deal of individual difference in reactions to sensory and perceptual deprivation among normal subjects.

These are a few of the many results of sensory deprivation studies on healthy young people. Depending on the type of reaction to sensory deprivation studied, the effects occurred within a few hours or a couple of days after onset of the experiment. If these reactions occurred so readily in normal, healthy persons, what would be the impact of sensory and perceptual restriction over a period of weeks or months on a person who has been severely injured? Thus, some of these data might be considered to be base rates for the occurrence of psychological disruption in restricted sensory and perceptual states in patients with spinal cord injury.

Consequently, the immediate reactions to spinal cord injury should be examined in terms of the psychological reactions to the physical aspects of the injury itself and the procedures utilized to assure the survival of the person. For example, the paralysis itself restricts movement and the procedures used to immobilize the spine will further restrict movement for at least eight weeks. Persons with quadriplegia, who have tongs in their head to immobilize the neck, have less movement possible than persons with paraplegia, and, furthermore, they have a more restricted visual field. They can look at the ceiling or the floor.

Medications to relax the person, to ease the pain, to treat associated problems, may cloud the sensorium for weeks after onset of the disability. It is not unusual for high dosages of muscle relaxants to be given to control muscle spasms later in the course of the disability; this can reduce mental acuity. Furthermore, anesthesia for surgery followed by treatment in intensive care units can produce a deterioration in the quality of mental functioning.

In intensive care units, there is little opportunity to rest comfortably because of the frequent interruptions required for medical procedures. In fact, for many months the person with spinal injury will be awakened every two hours in order to be turned to prevent skin lesions. Continued loss of sleep will disrupt mental efficiency further. There are few cues to identify the passage of time (often no windows, and lights on all the time), and, thus, disorientation for time and place could occur.

Loss of sensation associated with the injury is one form of sensory deprivation; the restricted view of the world (ceiling or floor) while in traction is another form of sensory deprivation. The monotony of the hospital routine is certainly a perceptual restriction, in addition to the lack of intellectual challenge which accompanies all long hospitalizations.

Pain may interfere with focused thinking and it may be a worry to the patient. Also, there are many hospital personnel who are doing many things *to* the person with spinal injury, much of which he may not understand at that point. He knows that he has been badly injured and he must trust those around him. If he does not trust them or if he is worried about it, he has essentially no choice. These procedures will continue to occur as the hospital system swings into action in order to ensure his survival.

Thus, one of the anxieties in this early stage after spinal injury may result from lack of information about what is happening. Harris and associates (1973) believe that patients and their families should be told at an early stage that paralysis is present and mention the implications for the immediate future. This information should be given by a member of the senior staff, but certainly not on the first day after injury. Braakman, Orbaan, and Dishoeck (1976) interviewed 60 persons with traumatic spinal injury who had been admitted to their hospital within six hours of the accident and asked them when they would have wished to receive the information about their condition. The authors found that 7 percent wanted the information on admission, 33 percent wanted to be told ''as soon as possible,'' 18 percent within the second week after injury. Thus, it appears that 58 percent of their sample wanted to understand their condition within two weeks of injury. Twenty-five percent said that the timing of the information depended on the mental status of the patient. These data suggest that persons with spinal cord injury tend to want to know what has happened to them and the implications for the future. However, there are individual differences in the patients' desire for information, and, thus, no hard and fast rule should be developed until we have more information as to whether the timing, the manner, or the amount of information influences the rehabilitation process.

Caywood (1974), in a description of his early experiences as a quadriplegic, makes a plea that the information about the disability be given in such a manner that it does not destroy the patient's hope that things might get better. He believes that this hope need not interfere with the rehabilitation process but can provide the strength to keep working despite the many frustrations of a rehabilitation program. He believes, and we concur, that hope is not necessarily the same as denial of disability and should not be placed in the same category as a defense mechanism.

A review of the literature on the psychological reactions to the early stages of spinal cord injury indicates that there is more speculation than fact contained in the few articles that deal with the acute stage. On the one hand, there is the paradigm that the early reaction is characterized by a massive denial process to prevent the person from facing the sudden changes in his body and the implications for the future. On the other hand, there is the paradigm proposed here that the immediate psychological reactions could be called ''normal reactions to an abnormal situation'' (Hohmann 1975), characterized by anxiety, reduction in mental acuity, and a somewhat clouded sensorium in reaction to the immobilization, altered and reduced sensory inputs, pain, drugs, and sleep disruption that are by-products of the efforts to keep the person alive after the accident. In any one person, either or both of these paradigms might account for the behavior in varying degrees. Both of these paradigms should be researched within the context of a respect for individual differences. Furthermore, it is hypothesized that the population of persons with spinal cord injury is a heterogeneous one and that the immediate reactions to the disability will be as varied as the preinjury personalities.

PROCESSES OF ADJUSTMENT TO SPINAL CORD INJURY

Are There Stages to the Adjustment Process?

The literature on the adjustment to spinal cord injury or physical disability in general is mixed as to whether there are stages to the adjustment to this injury. There are a fair number of publications that describe *the* stages to the adjustment process, but they vary as to how explicitly they state that these are the stages through which everyone goes. Several publications discuss the psychological problems of persons with spinal injury without explicitly stating that these are stages in the adjustment process; yet they seem to imply that all persons with spinal injury will exhibit these difficulties at some time. And there are a fair number of publications (many very recent) that emphasize the tremendous variability in the response to spinal cord injury and that challenge the stage theory of adjustment.

Wittkower and associates (1954) state that denial of disability is the first response to spinal cord injury. As noted above, however, the authors seem to equate the defense mechanism of denial with the patients' hope that they might get better. These authors go on to state that "in the early months of their disablement all patients, without exception, showed deep depression" (Wittkower et al. 1954, p. 111). They note that there were no functional psychoses in their group and only one case of psychoneurosis, and that in each of their 50 cases there was an intensification of the basic personality structure. Unfortunately, the tenor of the article is somewhat melodramatic, although it represents one of the early discussions of the psychosocial responses to spinal injury after World War II.

Dembo, Leviton, and Wright (1975) studied a group of amputees and wrote a treatise on the adjustment to misfortune. They describe the changes that are necessary in order for the person to accept the loss (defined as not devaluing oneself), and it seems implicit that these changes would be required of everyone who experiences a major loss. The changes include: enlarging the scope of values, containing the disability effects, subordinating physique, and transforming comparative values into asset values. The concept of mourning of the loss was introduced, and it is the resolution of the mourning by making the above changes that leads to adjustment to the disability. This theory was described by Wright (1960) who stated, "There is good reason to believe that the period of mourning can be a healing period during which the wound is first anesthetized and then gradually closed, leaving the least scarring" (Wright 1960, p. 114). Wright did caution, however, that this theory requires experimental verification before it can be accepted.

Siller (1969) states that anxiety and depression are the foremost reactions to physical traumatization and are readily observable. He cautions that if the superficial clinical picture suggests an absence of anxiety and depression, a more thorough observation will usually reveal their presence. If a recently disabled person does not seem particularly depressed, this is inappropriate. "A person should be depressed because something significant has happened, and not to respond as such is denial" (Siller 1969, p. 292). Siller further believes that grief and mourning behavior are necessary to the adjustment process; too speedy a rehabilitation program through the use of operant techniques, for example, may be counterproductive and interfere with the "work of mourning." This is tantamount to reinforcing a pattern of denial.

Kerr and Thompson (1972) feel that there are three stages in the adjustment process but present no data to substantiate their claims. The first stage is mental shock, fear, and anxiety, followed by a second stage of grief and mourning. Aggression and rebellion are the components of the third stage and are necessary in order to progress toward maturity. They imply that these stages are necessary for everyone in order to achieve good mental adjustment to the spinal cord injury. The remainder of their paper presents data on the variables associated with good versus poor mental adjustment following spinal injury, but Kerr and Thompson do not relate this data to their introductory statement about stages. The relationship is merely an inferential one, unsubstantiated by any data.

Berger and Garrett (1952) do not believe that all persons with paraplegia react to the disability in the same way; different persons, they assume, react to a disability in their own typical manner. However, they assert that certain behaviors occur frequently, e.g., depression, anxiety, and immature emotional expressions characterized by impulsiveness, explosiveness, and egocentric behavior. In addition, autistic or unrealistic thinking regarding the problems of life may be observed, along with a tendency toward ambivalence and indecision characterized by passive, submissive, and dependent behavior. Thus, having stated that people react differently, they then cite typical behaviors. This seems to be a contradiction.

Mueller (1962a) states that the initial reaction to spinal cord injury is depression, dependency, autistic thinking, and frustration.

The paraplegic tends to lack good human identification or empathy. He responds primarily to emotional elements of his environment and is easily motivated by external stimuli. His most prevalent emotional pattern is one of adolescent egocentricity, and there are many elements of uncontrolled infantile affective behavior. There is much uncontrolled emotionality and potential explosiveness. (Mueller 1962, pp. 152-53)

However, within three to six months, the person's preinjury personality reasserts itself. Thus, he believes that all persons with spinal injury react in a unitary fashion to the disability despite differences in preinjury styles of coping with stress. Unfortunately, his description of the reaction to disability makes the person with spinal injury seem like a Frankenstein.

Roberts (1972) proposes that all patients show some degree of "ego decompensation" as the result of the sudden onset of disability and states that symptoms of withdrawal, denial, or depression may be present.

Hohmann (1975) postulates that the normal person experiences a sequence of predominant feelings and attitudes as he attempts to cope with his injury. These are the normal sequelae to any severe loss and might be called "normal reactions to an abnormal situation." The first reaction is denial which lasts for three weeks to two months following injury. Relinquishing the mechanisms of denial ordinarily ushers in the reaction of depression. The first phase of the depressive reaction may be characterized by withdrawal and internalized hostility. Next, he externalizes the hostility onto those around him. And finally there is a reaction against dependence. After these reactions have been worked through, there will usually be a reconstitution of the preinjury personality, but there does not appear to be any personality type or trait associated with the disability. Rather there is an intensification of the preinjury traits.

Gunther (1969), using a psychoanalytic paradigm, presents a theoretical framework of the behavior change process following spinal cord injury. The first stage is shock, characterized by slow thought processes, some confusion, flat affect, and a reduced responsivity to the magnitude of the trauma. Partial recognition is the second stage, in which the person is more responsive to the environment but still protects himself against the feelings about his changed physical status. Initial stabilization, the next stage, is characterized by a shallow awareness of the existence of his lesion, and a superficial acceptance of it. Shock lasts hours or days, partial recognition lasts days to weeks, and initial stabilization lasts months or years. During this latter stage, the person appears cooperative and cheerful; his mood, mental processes, and capacity for interrelationships appear stable and appropriate. However, lest we think that all is well, Gunther cautions that this emotional adjustment is deceptive and will be followed by regression, anxiety, denial, and depression. Social recovery is the last stage in Gunther's theoretical framework.

Cull and Hardy (1977) assert that the person goes through the stages of adjustment described by Gunther, and, in addition, these authors utilize every one of the traditional defense mechanisms to describe the behavior of the person with spinal cord injury: denial, withdrawal, regression, repression, reaction formation, fantasy, rationalization, projection, identification, and compensation.

It is important to note that each of the preceding descriptions of stages of adjustment is based on the *clinical impressions of the particular author, and that no data have been presented in any of these articles to document the existence, sequence, or duration of these stages.* Hohmann (1975) states and others concur (Berger and Garrett 1952; Wright 1960; Shontz 1971) that there is no evidence of a unitary spinal cord injury personality type. Hohmann points out that the preinjury personality will reassert itself after these stages are worked through. Yet, one must ask, if there are many personality styles among persons with spinal cord injury, why must one assume that all will react to the onset of a disability in the same manner? Why must we assume that the injury will lead to a suspension of one's typical pattern of responding for a period of three to six months?

The "requirement of mourning" is described by Wright (1960) as the hypothesis that: "When a person has a need to safeguard his values, he will either 1) insist that the person he considers unfortunate is suffering (even when he seems not to be suffering) or 2) devaluate the unfortunate person because he ought to suffer and he does not" (Wright 1960, pp. 242-43). Wright also describes the "requirement of mourning" as the need to perceive the succumbing aspects rather than the coping aspects of living with a disability. In addition, she says that there may be an expectation discrepancy between the way the disabled person behaves and the way we expect him to behave. This happens because of the spread of effect.

> He (the observer) may, for example, *alter the apparent reality* by doubting the evidence concerning the adequate adjustment of the person with a disability. Thus, he may feel that the person is shamming, simply acting *as though* he were managing, when actually he is not. He (the observer) may suppress evidence regarding the coping aspect of difficulties and high-light evidence bearing upon the succumbing aspects. . . . (Wright 1960, pp. 73-74)

Is it possible that some of the publications that professionals have written reflect the "requirement of mourning"? Have professionals seen more distress and psychological difficulty than actually is present? Have professionals *uncritically* applied terms and theoretical concepts from the field of "mental illness" to describe the "normal reaction to an abnormal situation" which onset of spinal injury represents? Have professionals been describing phenomena that do not exist? Have professionals, in clinical interactions, placed disabled persons in a "Catch 22" position? If you have a disability, you must have psychological problems; if you state that you have no psychological problems, then this is denial and that is a psychological problem. And because of this, have psychologists, psychiatrists, social workers, and rehabilitation counselors lost credibility with other rehabilitation personnel and with persons who have spinal injury, and correctly so?

The stage theory of adjustment should be tested and longitudinal research procedures are the only legitimate approach to answer some of these questions. Such research should include a sufficiently large sample and the plans for data analysis should include procedures to assess the homogeneity versus heterogeneity of the sample studied. Such research should utilize direct measures of behavior, including a biochemical measure of emotion, rather than only the ratings or subjective impressions of rehabilitation personnel.

There has been a partial test of the stage theory of adjustment to spinal injury by Dunn (1969) who proposed to study seven psychological variables (role identity, ego strength, reality contact, rigidity, depression, self-concept, and anxiety) during three phases of rehabilitation (early, transitional, and late). He used the 16 Personality Factor Test as his measure of these variables and administered it twice with a four-week interval between tests. His sample consisted of 25 persons of all ages with spinal cord injury. None of his hypotheses of change were supported by the data, and the most striking result was the tremendous variability among the patients. Although this study could not be considered to be a rigorous test of the stage theory of adjustment to disability, it must be commended for its attempt to document a theory that has been accepted as true without question.

As long ago as 1950, Nagler described seven different types of reaction to spinal cord injury. His observations were based on a sample of 500 persons. He found: anxiety and reactive depression, psychotic reaction, indifference, psychopathic reaction, dependency reaction, reaction of the quadriplegic patient, and normal reaction. It is unfortunate that Nagler did not give frequency estimates for these categories, especially for the normal reaction group. Although Nagler's descriptions are as impressionistic as those cited by the stage theorists and are in terms associated with "mental illness," he does recognize the possibility of different types of reaction depending upon preinjury personality style.

The onset of spinal cord injury is not a minimal event in one's life, yet many persons with spinal injury state that it is not the most important thing that has ever happened to them. However, it must be a most unpleasant experience and one that a person would prefer to avoid if one had the choice. But it seems clear that professionals have stressed the negative emotional aspects unnecessarily and underestimated the strengths and coping ability of people in crisis.

Goldiamond (1973) describes some of his reactions to his own spinal injury and to the rehabilitation environment in an interesting article that is recommended to all who work with persons with spinal injury.

> When the professional refers to a patient as being "unaware of," "not realistic about," or "repressing" his problem, it is often the professional who is being unrealistic. If I choose not to discuss my pains, problems, and infections, it is not because I am unaware, unrealistic, or repressing. At times, I am painfully aware of them, and I mean that literally. If a patient does not "face up" to these issues, it may be because he is facing, or trying to face, in a different direction, one that can help him achieve his goals.
>
> Reaction to one's own injury is supposed to cause depression. By considering apathy, depression, or aggression as inevitable developmental stages in injury (or aging or illness), the professional staff can avoid asking how their actions might have been causal. (Goldiamond 1973, p. 100)

Depression versus Denial after Spinal Cord Injury

Dr. George Hohmann describes his reaction to spinal cord injury in these terms:

Patients today may not be as depressed as patients were 20 to 30 years ago. When I was injured 32 years ago, I was jolly well depressed, as I look back on it, because I was told that I would be dead in two years. I was told that I would never marry. I was told that I would never have a family. I was told that I would be in an institution for the remainder of my life, and the expectations were set by the institution and by the then prevailing knowledge. Today, patients are given, even in the very worst of centers, a very different type of expectation. It may be that the depression in 1977 is very different than it used to be. The intrapsychic sequelae may be very different in 1977 than they were in 1944. (Professional Conference 1977)

The information that a person with a recent spinal injury receives today is very different from that given in 1944. In the context of being told about the damage to his spinal cord and the prognosis for recovery, the physician will usually explain, in quite a bit of detail, the opportunities for leading a fairly normal life and outline the benefits of the rehabilitation program planned for the next several months. Although most persons will not be happy at the news about their physical status, the hope has been planted that they will not have to remain totally helpless forever. Perhaps, as Dr. Hohmann speculated, the intrapsychic sequelae are different today than in 1944. We will not be able to test this concept of changes in amount of depression in the last 30 years, but we can look carefully at the evidence that is accumulating about depression and denial in response to spinal cord injury today.

Bourestom and Howard (1965) compared the Minnesota Multiphasic Personality Inventory (MMPI) profiles of three disability groups, rheumatoid arthritis, multiple sclerosis, and spinal cord injury. They found that the group with spinal cord injury had the most benign profile, suggesting less emotional distress, the least anxiety, and least concern with somatic problems. Characterological defects often ascribed to such persons were not substantiated by the results. The average MMPI profile was entirely within normal limits and had little elevation of the ''neurotic triad'' in comparison with the other two groups.

Taylor (1967) studied a group of persons with spinal cord injury within a month of injury on the average and described the MMPI profiles of this group. The profiles were similar to that of a random sample of male university students with evidence of only very mild depression. There was no evidence of marked depression, anxiety, or psychotic mentation in his sample.

The concept of averaging MMPI profiles will be discussed in a later section as will other striking evidence from Taylor's study; however, it would appear that, as a group, on an objective test of depression, denial, and anxiety, persons with spinal cord injury do not fit the descriptions given in the literature describing the extreme psychological reaction to such injury.

Caywood (1974) did describe some stages in his early adjustment to quadriplegia but in very different terms than the professional literature reviewed in the previous section. His adjustments were:

1. Having no choice as to what was being done to his body

2. Realizing that it was his responsibility to put family, friends, and visitors at ease
3. Learning how to deal with people who appeared to be uncomfortable around him
4. Learning to rely on assistance with the most minor physical function
5. Becoming accustomed to the "relative indifference" of the staff once he moved to the rehabilitation center because he was no longer a special case
6. Realizing the extensiveness of the work ahead of him which the early days in therapy revealed
7. Coping with the tremendous fatigue at the end of each day of therapy
8. Not quitting in the face of frustration because everything was an effort and progress for a person with quadriplegia was so slow
9. Learning to assess his progress by the comments of visitors who had not seen him for a while.

It is interesting to note that Caywood does not mention depression per se in his description of his rehabilitation experiences.

Goldiamond believes that

> when depression does arise in the ill or disabled, it may be because consequences which used to be critical maintainers of behavior are no longer available, or the cost of obtaining these consequences may suddenly have become very high. A solution is to program actively either alternative consequences or alternative behavior patterns.
>
> This viewpoint leads us to reinterpret the nature of a patient's symptoms. The question is, what contingencies are now governing the patient's behavior? Far from indicating pathology, the patient's behavior may actually be the most sensible one possible, given the particular reinforcement contingencies in effect. (Goldiamond 1973, p. 100)

To achieve some clarity on the issue of depression, it is important to determine which definition of depression is being used at any one time since there is not unanimity on this point. Kolb (1973) believes that classical depression has its roots in unconscious guilt arising from interpersonal issues, perhaps unconscious anbivalence or hostility toward significant others in our environment. The hostile impulses originally directed toward the other person are directed toward oneself. Grief is to be differentiated from depression, however, according to Kolb, and is the affect of sadness suffered from a loss of something or someone important. Although leading to withdrawal and self-preoccupation, it is self-limiting.

Fordyce (1971) and Lazarus (1968) define depression or grieving as a deprivation of reinforcers. The sudden shift in the lifestyle of the person with spinal injury results in the termination or loss of those reinforcers in the environment that had sustained his behavior. Lazarus (1968) believes that when a significant reinforcer is withdrawn, the person enters a state of grief which lifts when he recognizes and utilizes other reinforcers at his disposal. Fordyce (1971) proposes that the effectiveness of a rehabilitation program will be related to the degree to which it arranges reinforcers that are relevant to the disabled person and contingent upon learning the behaviors specified in the rehabilitation program.

However, Seligman sees a similarity between the onset of depression and the development of learned helplessness. "Our theory of helplessness suggests that it is not the loss of reinforcers, but the loss of control over reinforcers, that causes depression" (Seligman 1975, p. 96). The depressed person believes or has learned that he cannot control those elements of his life that relieve suffering, bring gratification, or provide nurture. Thus, he believes that he is helpless.

In Seligman's theory, it is the belief in one's own inability to control the relevant reinforcers in one's life that becomes a critical issue in the depression. And people, because of their previous learning history, vary in their susceptibility to this belief. Those with a history of extensive experience in controlling and manipulating the sources of reinforcement in their lives should be more resistant to depression than those whose lives have been full of experiences in which they were helpless to influence the sources of their suffering. This formulation is consistent with Rotter's (1966) concept of internal versus external locus of control of reinforcement which will be discussed later. One other group of people are susceptible to depression, according to Seligman, and these are people who have experienced long histories of noncontingent reward. He believes that there is a certain segment of our youth who have had lives of complete reinforcement no matter what they did and, thus, they have never had the opportunity to learn a contingency between their behavior and the presence or absence of reinforcement. The book by Medved and Wallechinsky, *What Really Happened to the Class of '65* (1976), gives an illustration of this phenomenon.

Costello (1972) challenges the concept of depression as the loss of reinforcers and believes that depression is caused by the loss of reinforcer effectiveness. This loss of effectiveness is caused by: (1) endogenous biochemical and neurophysiological changes, and/or (2) the disruption of a chain of behavior, one kind of disruption being the loss of one of the reinforcers in the chain. He specifically avoids discussing the manner in which biochemical factors result in a loss of reinforcer effectiveness but cites data on the relative or absolute decrease in norepinephrine available at brain receptor sites during depression.

Each of these definitions of depression may increase our understanding of the reaction to spinal cord injury. The onset of the disability does, by definition, deprive one of a certain proportion of the rewards that had been important to the person, and one of the definitions of the impact of the disability is the degree of loss or change in previous lifestyle required by the disability. The early phases of the treatment of spinal cord injury certainly place the person in a helpless position, at least initially for persons with paraplegia, and for extended periods of time for persons with quadriplegia. Thus, a person could be susceptible to the belief that he could no longer control rewards and satisfactions in his life. Variations in this susceptibility may be related to previous life circumstances and, thus, the factor of internal versus external locus of control may determine one's reaction to the experience of being helpless. Using Kolb's differentiation, grief seems to be a more appropriate label to apply to the reaction to spinal cord injury than classical depression. However, it is obvious that these multiple connotations of depression complicate the issue of reaction to disability and, in future research, care must be taken to specify the definition of depression.

There have been a number of interesting studies into the incidence of depression after onset of spinal cord injury. Klas (1970) did a longitudinal study of four persons with quadriplegia and found that there was no consistent relationship between depression and performance in therapies and that the staff usually rated patients as more depressed than the patients' self-ratings. Although the measurement of depression in this study could have been more rigorous and the small number of cases complicates the interpretation of these results, an intensive study of patients over time in order to assess the flow of behavior has much to recommend it.

Kalb (1971) studied the relationship between noncooperative and depressive behavior during hospitalization and 11 posthospital behaviors in 24 white males with spinal injury. He found that middle socioeconomic status (SES) subjects showed a significant and *positive* correlation between degree of ward noncooperation and the range of posthospital behaviors and that degree of depression was not related to any of the outcome variables. However, for lower SES subjects, the greater the depression, the poorer the performance on the outcome variables, and ward noncooperation was unrelated to all outcome variables except school and employment in which case more noncooperation was associated with poorer performance in this area. Social class by itself was not a good predictor of noncooperation or depression in the hospital or of posthospital behavior. But when knowledge of SES was combined with knowledge of hospital behavior, predictions could be made about posthospital behavior. Furthermore, all low SES patients who received high noncooperation scores had a preinjury history of difficulty adjusting to society. This was not the case for middle SES subjects.

Dinardo (1971) performed an excellent study of the thesis that absence of depression does not necessarily imply denial of disability and subsequent maladjustment. Rather, individuals whose emotional response styles predispose them to depression as a reaction to spinal injury will have greater difficulty in adjusting to the disability than those who do not display such a response style. He studied 26 persons with spinal cord injury in terms of their locus of control and tendency to be a repressor or a sensitizer in emotional situations. He found that internals have higher self-concepts than externals, and externals are more depressed than internals. Also, internal repressors show the best adjustment to spinal cord injury, and external sensitizers show the poorest adjustment. Absence of depression favored good adjustment. In fact, those who reacted with depression were less well adjusted at any given point in their rehabilitation than individuals who did not react with depression. Thus, he concluded that there was no evidence that absence of depression was equated with denial of illness or portended maladjustment.

In an extension of this line of research, Lawson (1976, 1978) wondered if there is a period of depressive affect or grief following spinal cord injury and whether there are any events in the rehabilitation process associated with depressive or elative affect. Ten persons with quadriplegia were studied longitudinally five days a week for their entire length of hospital stay (average of 119 days). Each patient dictated a nightly record (what, when, with whom, emotional reactions) of each day's events into a portable tape recorder. He had four measures of depressive affect: daily self-report to a semantic differential by the patient, behavioral measure of the number of words per minute during the first three minutes of their daily taping session, daily average of semantic differentials rated by four staff members, endocrine measure of daily output of urinary tryptamine. He found that there were no clear periods of depressive affect; no patient had extended depressive periods in which 70 percent of the measures were in the depressive range. There were significant individual differences for each measure of depressive affect. Nevertheless, the scores of these patients with quadriplegia were similar in average and range to scores for normal (nondepressed) persons.

He found that the period two to three weeks after admission was the most depressive period on all four measures and the period just before discharge was characterized by significant depressive and elative reactions. In addition, the patients who were least depressed during the hospital phase performed best on two measures of posthospital adjustment and the person who was most depressed had died.

Lawson's study must be complimented for its comprehensiveness: the multiple levels of measurement of depression and the longitudinal and intensive analysis of the behavior of ten persons with spinal injury. Therefore, it should serve as a model of the type of research that must be conducted in this field.

Consequently, it appears that we might tentatively conclude that spinal injury *does not* lead to severe depressive reactions in all patients and the absence of depression does not seem to imply denial of illness or poor adjustment to disability. On the average, mild depression might be present depending on the type of measure used; therefore, the need for multiple levels of measurement of depression has been amply demonstrated by Lawson's study. Each study noted the individual differences in emotional response to the disability which is further evidence for the heterogeneity of the population with spinal injury.

It is interesting to note the differences in depressive reaction according to SES in Kalb's study. If we assume that those persons who have a history of learning that they are unable to control any rewards in their life to relieve their suffering and gain satisfaction are more predisposed to depression, as professed by Seligman (1975), then these persons fit the description of those with an external locus of control. Lefcourt (1966, 1976) points out that persons with a low SES are likely to score as externals on measures of locus of control. Thus, the factors of locus of control and SES should be evaluated in future studies in this area.

Dinardo's study confirmed the notion that locus of control is relevant to the issue of depressive reactions and, in addition, found that those who express their depressive feelings are less likely to do well.

Are internals less depressed than externals or do they "cover it up" or express it differently? Lawson's study included a self-report, a behavioral measure, a staff rating, and an endocrine measure of depression. It would be interesting to test internals and externals on these multiple measures, especially including a biochemical measure to assess this question.

Klas found that depressive behavior was associated with low levels of positive reinforcement. However, we do not know if there is a causative effect, and, if so, in which direction. When the patients were depressed, did they display fewer behaviors that could be positively reinforced or did they receive less positive reinforcement because of variations in therapist behavior and then become depressed? We do not know.

Studies of psychoendocrine function emphasize the importance of including such measures in future studies on the emotional reactions to disability. Bunney, Mason, and Hamburg (1965) studied urinary 17-Hydroxycorticosteroids (17-OHCS) in psychiatrically hospitalized depressed patients and found that depression correlates more with 17-OHCS than does anxiety. However, the heterogeneity of patient response was again noted. High positive significant correlations were found between depression and 17-OHCS when serial determinations were run over time for a given patient. But, if mean depression rating and mean corticosteroid level were taken on each patient, a significant correlation was not obtained. Thus, again we see the need for longitudinal studies with successive measures on the same patients. Cross-sectional studies using one or several measures may not be sufficient to understand emotional reactions.

McDaniel and Sexton (1970) studied 22 males, recently injured, with lesions at L_1 to T_7. Four periods in the hospitalization were preselected for their potential stressfulness (admission, learning transfers, ambulation, and discharge) and behavioral ratings by staff and plasma cortisol and catecholamine excretion measures were obtained at each of these four time periods. The behavior ratings differed significantly across periods, with admission and discharge seeming to be the most stressful. However, ratings of depression, irritability, and use of denial remained constant over time. The biochemical data are less clear. There was a significant difference in these measures across the four periods, but there was no significant interaction between any periods.

Looking at previous studies and the heterogeneity of response noted, it is probable that any differences in emotional response among the subjects negated each other. For example, there are only four measures on each subject and these were obtained at times that McDaniel and Sexton labeled as stressful, rather than using Lawson's more empirical approach of having a stressful period defined according to the behavioral response of the subject. Furthermore, as indicated by the above studies, persons vary in their response to spinal cord injury, but McDaniel and Sexton were looking for average reaction. Their subjects were also less disabled than subjects with high thoracic and cervical lesions. Therefore, it is difficult to draw any conclusions from this study. However, it does point out that intermittent biochemical measures will not be as helpful as serial determination on the same patient.

Hohmann (1966) conducted structured interviews with 25 males with spinal injuries at varying levels and asked them to compare their emotional feelings before and after their injury. He found that persons with cervical and high thoracic lesions reported a marked reduction in feelings of sexual stimulation, fear, and anger. In persons with lower thoracic and lumbar lesions, there was a moderate to mild reduction in these feelings. Almost all persons reported an increase in feelings of sentimentality since their accident. Although these men reported a reduction of experienced emotional feeling, they tended to continue to display overt evidence of emotion because the environment seemed to expect it of them. In addition, it usually helped them get what they wanted. Thus, they tended to act more emotional than they actually felt. These results were interpreted as evidence that disruption of the autonomic nervous system and its afferent return causes notable changes in experienced emotional feelings.

The Hohmann study should be replicated because the results could have wide-ranging significance in terms of emotional reaction to spinal injury. However, Hohmann not only generated the hypothesis of reduced emotionality but was the interviewer of the subjects; thus, the opportunity for experimental bias is present. Several persons with spinal injury have disputed these results, including one person who was a subject in the study. One wonders, therefore, if there might be another interpretation for these results.

The study was conducted in the late 1950s when the average length of hospitalization was in terms of years, not months, and the message communicated to the spinal injured person was less encouraging than at present. Perhaps the subjects had learned to suppress many of their feelings (except for sentimentality, interestingly) as a means of coping with a discouraging and depressing reality. Even today persons with spinal injury report that they have to learn to *minimize* the difficulties of living with a disability as a means of coping with the daily frustrations, the prejudice and thoughtlessness of able-bodied persons, and the hard work of everyday survival. In fact, several persons with quadriplegia have reported that it would be great if they could occasionally take a vacation from being a "quad."

Yet, if the Hohmann results are substantiated by further research, the concept of a reduced ability to experience emotions is quite discomforting to many persons with spinal injury. They tend to fear that this would make them less of a human being, less of a person than they used to be. Perhaps one of the key factors in coping with a physical disability may be the assurance that one gives oneself that it is only the physical body that is different, but the human being, the personality, remains the same.

Hohmann's results suggesting that disruption of the autonomic nervous system influences experienced emotional feelings may provide some fascinating and exciting avenues for research. A review of neuroanatomy reveals that pathways of enervation of the viscera and other bodily parts associated with the physiological aspect of emotion are located in the spinal cord and transection of the cord would indeed block cortical perception of these sensations. Schachter (1971) has studied emotion for a number of years and proposes that the experience of an emotion is a function of a state of physiological arousal and a cognitive interpretation of this arousal state. This leads to the following hypotheses: given a state of physiological arousal for which the person has no immediate explanation, he will "label" the state and describe his feelings according to the cognitions available to him; given a state of physiological arousal for which the person has an appropriate explanation, he will not label his feelings in terms of alternative cognitions available; given the same cognitive circumstances, the individual will act emotionally or describe his feelings as emotions only to the extent that he experiences a state of physiological arousal.

Schachter cites the Hohmann (1966) study as evidence in favor of his third hypothesis. In addition, he cites research demonstrating that physiological arousal facilitates the learning of an avoidance behavior or an emotional behavior, and, after a sympathectomy (excision of a portion of the autonomic nervous system), this avoidance or emotional behavior will be maintained. However, after a sympathectomy, the learning of a new avoidance response or emotional behavior will be significantly impaired according to certain animal research. What, then, are the implications for learning to avoid pressure sores or other medical problems in persons with spinal injury who have suffered a sympathectomy as a result of spinal cord injury?

If Hohmann's data and Schachter's theory of emotion are correct, then following a spinal injury, a person would seem depressed and would certainly have the cognitions that one associates with depression, but he may not feel the depression to the same degree as prior to the accident. Yet Hohmann reports a slight increase in feelings of sentimentality. Whether this means that depressive feelings are uninterrupted by autonomic nervous system disruption or whether this implies a greater appreciation of warm, tender, or other interpersonal experiences after surviving a catastrophic injury, we do not know.

However, if persons with spinal injury tend to act "as if" they were emotional because of the cues they receive from their enviornment, we must be very cautious in our experimental designs. Multiple levels of measurement will be necessary; longitudinal assessments will be necessary; data analyses that examine individual differences will be necessary; specification of severity of injury will be necessary; use of control groups of others who have suffered a catastrophic insult but whose autonomic nervous system remained intact will be necessary. Thus, research into the emotional aspects of disability must become more sophisticated and should begin to test some of the myths that have remained unquestioned for years.

In essence, however, these studies indicate that depression is not as severe nor as prevalent as had been suspected following spinal injury. Consequently, a more precise use of the term ''depression'' is advocated. Classically, depression is characterized by loss of appetite, insomnia, and psychomotor retardation, but depression in this sense does not occur to the majority of persons following spinal injury. Therefore, the term ''grief'' seems more appropriate to describe the sadness and loss one would feel when suddenly disabled. Many disabled persons report that the most ''depressing'' thing is the staff expectation that they should be ''depressed'' (Lawson 1977). Thus, it would appear that professionals consistently perceive more grief than the person actually experiences which may be a further example of able-bodied people imposing the ''requirement of mourning'' on disabled people.

The research tends to show that mourning the loss through a display of depressive behaviors is not necessary for adjustment to the disability. In fact, the contrary appears to be true. Those that truly and obviously mourn the loss in the manner that the professional literature demands appear to be coping less well; fortunately, they constitute a minority of the disabled population. Most persons with disabilities have significant strengths and coping ability, and this fact appears to have been seriously underestimated by many professionals. Furthermore, absence of depression does not imply a denial of the disability, denial being another term that has been used improperly.

Denial seems to occur in a very small proportion of persons who become suddenly disabled. It may be defined as the refusal to participate in any of the rehabilitation activities because these activities are perceived to be unnecessary. The person expects to recover completely and views rehabilitation as a waste of time. These cases are rare, but when they occur, discharge to the home environment after the family has been trained to prevent deterioration may be an appropriate course of action. The person can spend time in his or her own environment and observe whether or not recovery occurs. However, all efforts should be made to maintain contact with the person so that he or she can return for training at some later date if desired.

Sometimes hope of recovery or statements such as ''I am going to walk out of here'' are confused with denial. However, as long as the person is participating in the rehabilitation program, these statements become an understandable and natural reaction to sudden disability.

Other Factors in the Process of Adjustment to Spinal Cord Injury

Motivation. Motivation is a very complex topic and no attempt will be made to explore all parameters of this issue in depth. However, three approaches to the concept of motivation will be discussed since the treatment strategies will differ according to which approach is used. One approach considers motivation to be a dynamic force within the individual; one considers motivation to be those rewards in the environment for which the person will work; and one is a combination of these two, postulating that the individual's locus of control in interaction with environmental rewards will be the key to motivation.

Most rehabilitation specialists agree that a critical factor in the success of their professional efforts will be a motivated patient. Heijn (1971) states that mastery of the emotional task of accepting one's loss is necessary before one can become motivated to participate in the rehabilitation process. Heijn and Granger (1974) elaborate upon these ideas and believe that rehabilitation success or failure is often determined by cognitive and emotional factors, and the assessment and nurturing of these factors should receive the same degree of attention as do physical functions. They believe that patients who have motivational problems, which limit progress toward realization of expected potential in all aspects of treatment, can be identified by observing "differential motivation" in certain areas of rehabilitation. Occupational therapy is considered by them to be the barometer as to where the patient stands regarding resolution of the cognitive and emotional stresses of disability. If a patient is unable to mourn his loss and accept his disability, his motivation will remain low, they believe. Thus, these authors give advice on how to identify the presence and absence of motivation, and they discuss the importance of motivation to the rehabilitation process; they do not, however, describe what to do in the absence of motivation except to encourage the person to mourn his loss.

Diamond, Weiss, and Grynbaum (1968) state that successful physical rehabilitation demands a cooperative patient. Thus, they try to identify factors that differentiate participants from nonparticipants. Essentially they found that participants were positive, hopeful, and future-oriented and nonparticipants were negative, resigned, and past-oriented. They report, however, that in their experience, nonparticipants do not benefit from standard psychotherapy which is aimed at exploring the motivational deficit. Thus, they conclude that the problem of motivation must involve not only the patient but also the mutual interactions of patient and rehabilitation staff (the patient-environment interaction).

Rabinowitz (1961) outlined four hypotheses to differentiate between well-motivated and poorly motivated persons:

1. Realism and clarity of goal-striving ambitions.
2. Acceptance of suitable value-standards and behavior patterns.

3. Demonstration of adequate tolerance for frustration-producing experiences.
4. An increasing degree of autonomy as suggested by development of more egalitarian feelings toward hospital staff.

Implicity, Rabinowitz locates these four parameters within the individual but does recognize that the operation of a hospital as a social system will influence these variables.

Chanin and Brown (1975) evaluated the reasons that persons with spinal cord injury had been closed from plan (case closed before successful completion of the program) by the California State Department of Rehabilitation in 1972–1973. By counselors' reports, the two most frequently cited reasons for nonrehabilitation were the clients' lack of cooperation and follow-through. These reasons accounted for one-third of those cited.

The definition of motivation is not always specified in articles that discuss its importance, but frequently, it is synonymous with cooperation or compliance with rehabilitation staff goals for that patient. But Albrecht and Higgins (1977) in a fascinating study of the interrelationships of multiple criteria of rehabilitation success point out that motivation or cooperation in the rehabilitation setting does not accurately predict independent living after discharge. They found that cooperation and completion of services correlated from 0.07 to 0.23 with improvement in physical functioning. They also discovered that some patients who displayed the greatest independence (a purported goal of rehabilitation) were judged to be uncooperative by the staff and to have failed to complete the staff's conception of a rehabilitation program.

Ludwig and Adams (1968) studied the relationship between patient cooperation and completion of rehabilitation services. They hypothesized that successful completion of services requires the assumption of the client role and that some persons would assume this role more readily than others. Thus, they examined the background characteristics of those who completed and those who did not complete services. Those patients most likely to complete services were the very young and very old, females, nonwhites, unemployed, those sponsored by public agencies (except workman's compensation), and those with severe handicaps. They concluded that those whose normal role relationships and social position contained elements of dependency and subordination were more likely to successfully perform in the role of client and complete a treatment program.

Wendland (1973) was devising a scale in order to measure the cooperation among rehabilitation patients. However, one must ask whether cooperation is necessarily desirable if it has a low correlation with physical functioning and if it has a moderately high correlation with dependency or subordinate roles in society. It has yet to be demonstrated that cooperation with current rehabilitation procedures is the best measure of rehabilitation success.

All of these opinions focus upon motivation as a characteristic of the individual and relate it to the process of adjusting (mourning) to the disability. Motivation is often synonymous with cooperation with rehabilitation goals set by the staff for the patient without really involving the patient in the goal-setting process. None of these articles identifies effective remedies for those who lack motivation and, therefore, they emphasize the process of identification of the presence or absence of motivation.

However, Margolin (1971) believes that motivation is not the problem at all and that ''designating a patient as unmotivated is inaccurate, unrealistic, and a block to rehabilitation progress'' (Margolin 1971, p. 94). He believes that there are many environmental factors acting to help or hinder a person's progress, and he categorizes these as the hospital system, family system, social system, employment system, and school system. The hospital and family are the two most important systems affecting the patient's behavior and, according to Margolin, ''Physicians, nurses, therapists, spouses, and parents not infrequently are the primary causative agents contributing to the patient's failure syndrome'' (Margolin 1971, p. 96).

Goldiamond (1973, 1976) states that for him there was a direct contingency between participation in the rehabilitation program and the resumption of his professional activities which were very important to him. ''I believe that the existence or absence of such a relation was what distinguished those patients whom the hospital staff called 'motivated' from those they called ''unmotivated' '' (Goldiamond 1973, p. 97). When participation in the program had critical consequences for the patient, he participated.

In describing some of his fellow patients who showed minimal involvement in the rehabilitation program, he states:

Such cases puzzled the hospital staff. After all, people should *want* to get better, should *want* to stay alive longer. The staff knew how to make them better; so the patients should *want* to cooperate. When they did not, the staff would give them pep talks or scare talks, warning of the dire consequences of degeneration, show them movies, reason with them, etc. None of those tactics helped.

The staff ascribed the negative attitudes of such patients to hostility, depression, or some other underlying psychodynamic problem. But none of these labels were relevant to the real problem, namely, the absence of consequences important enough to sustain the difficult responses necessary for producing and maintaining them. (Goldiamond 1973, pp. 97–98)

For two very excellent descriptions of the reaction to disability from the behavioral point of view, the discussions by Michael (1970) and by Fordyce (1971) should be consulted. In essence, in behavioral terms, the onset of disability may be viewed as a punishment defined as either the loss of positive reinforcers or the onset of aversive stimuli. Both of these situations are characteristic of the initial phases of disability. However, punishment tends to increase the behaviors designed to avoid or escape the punishment and, thus, the rehabilitation therapies that entail facing the disability may be avoided. Fantasy and wishful thinking may be rewarded since they also avoid facing the disability. Thus, rehabilitation strategies would be directed toward decreasing the aversive features of the rehabilitation activities and decreasing the positive consequences of successful avoidance or escape behavior.

To accomplish this, Fordyce (1971) recommends that graded tasks be specified and scaled in order to maximize the probability of success, that rewards be identified and delivered for performance of these tasks, and that rate of reward should decrease and behavioral expectations should increase as progress occurs. A critical feature of this entire process is a good relationship between client and staff and active participation of the client in planning his own treatment program.

In contrast to some recommendations that the patient must be allowed to have time to mourn his loss, Fordyce recommends that withdrawal behaviors should be actively interrupted by presenting the client with specific rehabilitation tasks. Siller (1969), however, is quite worried that such procedures are counterproductive and interfere with successful adjustment to the disability. Thus, we have another question for future research.

Within the behavioral framework, one must specify what behaviors the person will need to cope with his own environment and identify rewards for which the person will work (Trieschmann 1974). Thus, lack of motivation means that there may be few rewards contingent on the occurrence of rehabilitation behaviors. The remedy is to alter the reward contingencies rather than to attempt to change the attitudes of the person. Motivation, then, becomes external to the person and can be influenced by the behaviors of each member of the rehabilitation team. If rehabilitation is the process of learning to live with one's disability in one's own environment, then each member of the rehabilitation team becomes a teacher and, thus, a rewarder or punisher of the patient's behavior. Consequently, as Margolin (1971) points out, the hospital staff are a critical element in the patient's motivation or reward system.

Lane and Barry (1970), in a review of the literature on client motivation in rehabilitation, state that the term "motivation" has been used to account for the causality in behavior precisely because all of the relevant variables were not known. They believe that because of the extreme complexity of human behavior, scientists have found it easier to postulate vaguely defined internal processes or motives in accounting for behavior than to search for precise relationships between antecedent variables and observed behaviors. Fordyce (1975), in his review of the literature on efforts to increase patient participation, concurs and believes that *success lies not in screening out marginally motivated persons but in an examination of and reprogramming of the interactions between patient behavior and environmental response or consequence.*

Learned helplessness. Seligman (1975) has conducted many excellent laboratory experiments to determine the effects on behavior of experiencing uncontrollable trauma. He has developed a theory of learned helplessness which states that a person becomes helpless when an outcome occurs that is independent of all of his voluntary responses. Thus, if a person is in an aversive, traumatic situation and he finds that nothing that he does will terminate the trauma, he experiences the feeling of helplessness, and his motivation to respond in the face of later trauma is reduced. The major consequences of experience with uncontrollable events are: (1) motivational: there is a reduced motivation to initiate voluntary responses that control other events; (2) cognitive: when a person has had the experience of uncontrollability, he has trouble learning that his new response has succeeded when it actually did, and thus there is a distortion of the perception of control; (3) emotional: initially there is a heightened state of emotionality (fear) which, with further experience with uncontrollability, changes to depression.

Seligman believes that directive therapy is the cure for learned helplessness. The individual must learn that there is again a contingency between his behavior and consequences in the environment. He must be actively taken through the responding process repeatedly so that he can have the experience that his behavior can control his environment. (This is similar to Fordyce's active interruption of withdrawal.)

Trieschmann (1975, 1976) has described the similarities between Seligman's experiments which produce learned helplessness and the early stages of spinal cord injury. She notes that the onset of spinal cord injury is a traumatic and highly aversive event and, in the first several weeks (much longer for persons with quadriplegia), the person is in fact helpless to control the events around him. No matter what the person does, the terrible event (treatment procedures for spinal injury and the deficits of the injury itself) remains a reality, and gradually some persons may cease making efforts to control the environment.

Wortman and Brehm (1975) discuss the evidence on learned helplessness in terms of reactance theory which states that when a person's behavioral freedom is threatened, he will become motivationally aroused. This motivational arousal, called reactance, leads individuals to try to restore their freedom. The amount of reactance that a person will display is a direct function of the expectation that he possesses the freedom in the beginning, the strength of the threat to his freedom, the importance of the freedom being threatened, and the implications of the threat for his other freedoms. In order to explain adequately Seligman's data, they argue, there must be an integration of reactance theory and learned helplessness theory.

Thus, they propose that when a person expects to control outcomes that are important to him and finds these outcomes uncontrollable, he will become aroused since this is a threat to his freedom. Initially, he will exert greater efforts to control the outcomes but eventually he learns that he, in fact, has no control. At that point he stops trying. Reactance should precede helplessness for persons who originally expect control. One would predict that the stronger the expectation of control, the longer it would take the person to become helpless. Those who do not expect to have control should not experience reactance and should become helpless relatively quickly.

However, Averill (1973) cautions that the relationship between personal control and stress is not simple. He believes that the only statement that can be made with assurance is that the stress-inducing or stress-reducing properties of personal control depend on the meaning of the control response for the individual, and what lends meaning to a response is the context in which it is embedded.

There is an interesting theme that occurs in the explanations of Seligman and Wortman and Brehm concerning learned helplessness: the heterogeneity of response and the expectancy of control. Seligman reports a study in which those persons who scored as externals in locus of control became helpless much more rapidly than the other subjects. Externals tend to believe that rewards and punishments occur through fate or chance and, thus, would not seem to believe that they have much control over events or outcomes. Wortman and Brehm point out that previous expectation of control over outcomes should determine how rapidly one succumbs to the feeling of helplessness. Thus, these speculations pose some interesting research questions for the future since the onset of spinal cord injury may be one of the most extreme examples of uncontrollability that occurs in the natural environment.

Internal versus external locus of control (I-E). Rotter (1966) hypothesizes that there are consistent individual differences among people in the degree to which they believe that they have personal control over reward. People who are external believe that the rewards or punishments in life occur as the result of chance, luck, fate, or powerful others. Internals, however, believe that rewards or punishments occur as the result of their own actions. The critical issue in this hypothesis is not the reality of the control over reward, but the person's learned belief or expectancy about the relationship between his behavior and outcomes. It is interesting to note that research has indicated that lower socioeconomic persons tend to score more frequently as externals and higher socioeconomic persons tend to score more frequently as internals (Lefcourt 1966, 1976).

Lefcourt (1966, 1976) provides an excellent review of the research findings on the I-E dimension, only some of which will be noted here. Consistent with Averill's (1973) observations about control and stress, Lefcourt notes that reactions to aversive stimuli are evidently shaped and molded by our perception of these stimuli and by our perception of our ability to cope with these stimuli. Those who are in a higher social position or group and who have greater access to valued outcomes are more likely to hold internal control expectancies. Internals are more likely to resist attempts to influence them on issues that conflict with their already established beliefs and values. Persons with an external orientation have learned that life's satisfactions and misfortunes are not highly related to their own behavior and are, thus, less apt to exert themselves or persist over time in trying to obtain distant goals. If tomorrow brings us possible calamity, why deny oneself today's small offerings of pleasure. Long-range efforts become absurd if we know that we will be encountering daily uncertainty, Lefcourt states. It should be noted, however, that there is some reason to believe that locus of control for success and for failure may be relatively independent of each other and, therefore, we should not necessarily expect a unidimensionality of the I-E phenomenon.

Internals tend to show less tension and depression than externals do and are more likely to remain active in their attempts to cope with crisis events. Seeman and Evans (1962) studied the I-E dimension in patients with tuberculosis in relation to the amount of knowledge they had about their disease. The results are discussed in terms of alienation. They found that high alienation persons (externals) had significantly lower scores on tests of objective knowledge about their disease. They state that knowledge acquisition is irrelevant for those who believe that fate, luck, or external forces control the fall of events.

Albrecht and Higgins (1977) found that locus of control scores became more internal as individuals progressed through their rehabilitation program. Meyerson (1968) studied the relationship between physical disability and sense of competence. He assumed that locus of control would be an adequate measure of sense of competence. Only one variable correlated significantly with the I-E score and that was race. Blacks were more external in their orientation than whites. Degree of disability did not correlate significantly with I-E.

Dinardo's (1971) study was described in detail in the section on depression. He found that internals were less depressed than externals and internals had better self-concepts than did externals. He concluded that response to spinal cord injury depended on preinjury personality style, that is, internal versus external locus of control.

Swenson (1976) did a follow-up study of persons with spinal injury and compared outcomes according to locus of control. He found that internals versus externals: spent less time in the hospital as the result of nonhygienic behaviors; were more satisfied with life; spent more time in work activities in the home, in educational activities, and in time outside of their home; and spent more time in some combination of educational activities, paid employment, and community work. In addition, his study did not find any correlation between severity of disability and I-E or satisfaction with life. Thus, even though a person with quadriplegia may in fact have less control over his immediate circumstances, this does not necessarily change the generalized expectancy of control over the rewards in life nor satisfaction with life.

An expanded view of motivation. Motivation is an important factor in the process of adjustment to spinal cord injury, and it has received considerable attention. However, it is a summary term which we use to describe all of those features that determine whether or not the person will incorporate the teachings of rehabilitation into his lifestyle. Traditionally, we have assumed that motivation is exclusively a characteristic of the person himself; recently, however, there has been an increasing amount of evidence to suggest that the definition of motivation as an internal drive state is too limited a view of the situation. Rather, we have evidence (presented in chapter 8) that the use of operant techniques on ''unmotivated'' persons changes their behavior so that it is similar to that of ''motivated'' persons. Thus, we have begun to look at the environment as a critical element in the assessment of the person's motivation. In this approach, the unmotivated person is the one for whom we have no reward for which he will work. The focus is external to the person and is on rewards and punishments in the environment.

However, Seligman has proposed that merely having a powerful reward available in the environment may not be sufficient if the person has learned that there is no contingency between his behavior and the outcomes. As has been previously discussed, he calls this learned helplessness. Indeed, this helpless state occurs as the result of the process of learning and can be corrected through the process of learning, but not without paying more attention to the person and what he brings with him into the learning situation. If a person has experienced a learned helplessness situation, such as the onset of spinal cord injury, for example, he may have an expectancy that there is nothing that he can do to influence the outcome. Thus, he may not emit the very first behavior that the behaviorists need in order to give him the reward. Seligman further states that even the experience of one reward or several does not necessarily change the person's expectancy that there is no relationship between his behavior and the outcomes.

There are individual differences in one's susceptibility to the learned help-lessness phenomenon, and the locus of control dimension may account for a significant part of the variance. Locus of control is an expectancy or set that one brings with one into a learning situation. This dimension of personality developed through the process of learning and was very much influenced by environmental rewards and punishments. Yet, once this dimension is learned, it may influence the number of occasions that are needed to produce helpless-ness (perhaps never in some internals); it may influence the type of reward, the schedule of reward, and the ability to delay reward in one person versus another.

Within the context of spinal cord injury, are externals more vulnerable to the learned helplessness phenomenon? Do externals need a more highly structured program than internals; in fact, is this necessary in order to get externals going? Do internals resent a highly structured program and do they function better when they define their own schedule and set their own behavioral goals? Do externals perform better with rewards specified for particular behaviors and are these more likely to be materialistic or primary rewards? Do internals find praise and charting of their own behavior to be sufficiently rewarding in order to progress through the rehabilitation process? Do we need to give greater attention to the postdischarge program (and, perhaps, structure it as much as possible) for externals since evidence suggests that they are more depressed and less involved in many activities following discharge?

Thus, it is proposed that progress in understanding the process of adjustment to spinal cord injury will not be made by looking only at the person as the seat of motivation and it will not be made by looking only at rewards and punishments available in the person's environment. Rather, future advances in the state of the art will require an integration of these two approaches.

Body Image

Body image is a term that refers to the body as a psychological experience and includes one's feelings and attitudes toward one's own body, body parts, and body functions. Traditionally, body image was viewed as necessary for the development of the total ego structure and was an important concept within psychoanalytic theory. Today, body image does not seem to be as popular a concept in personality theory as it was 20 or 30 years ago, but the onset of spinal cord injury does provoke interest in this issue. The literature on body image in spinal injury is limited, and the articles seem to fall into two categories: those written by neurologists describing distortions in perception of one's body following spinal injury, and those written by psychologists attempting to relate body image to disability adjustment.

Evans (1962) points out that if body image is defined as total awareness of one's body, then any injury that would interfere with this awareness would by definition disturb the body image. Body image, he believes, is composed of perceptual images derived from immediate sensory experience and from memory images derived from previous knowledge. The perceptual image of the body is dependent on two sources of sensory data, those providing information from outside the integument, chiefly visual or tactile from contact of one part with another, and those providing information wholly from within the body, tactile and kinesthetic. These would be termed external and internal sources of data. Thus, in spinal injury the internal source of information about body image is lost but external sources remain. In amputees, however, both sources of data are lost.

Bors (1951) studied 50 men with spinal injury and found that the incidence of body image distortions was 100 percent. However, in contrast to the body image distortions (phantom limb sensations) of amputees, those with spinal injury reported no telescoping or shrinkage of the phantom sensation over time. Heilporn and Noel (1968) report that several of their 40 cases of spinal injury experienced changes in body image, but they do not give much information.

Conomy (1973) does, however, describe the types of body image distortions that were experienced by his sample of 18 traumatically injured persons with spinal injury. He found that all of his persons with spinal injury showed at least some fragmentary disruption of the body scheme. Eighty-nine percent of his cases experienced a disordered perception of the body in space (proprioceptive body image). This distortion occurred early after the injury, for many of them at the moment of injury. The sensation of the legs being positioned in other than their visually perceived location persisted intermittently for lengthy periods (unspecified length of time). Perceptual distortions regarding the upper extremities occurred less frequently. The patients described the feeling of their legs floating upward from the bed, extended at the knees and ankles, and slightly flexed at the hips.

A second type of body image distortion reported was a disordered perception of posture or movement (disorders of kinetic body image). Seventy-two percent of his cases reported this effect, and it was described as a strong sense of muscular work with resulting fatigue. Disorders of perception of somatic bulk, size, and continuity (somatic body image) were reported in 39 percent of the cases. This disorder took the form of a hallucinated increase in the size of feet and legs. Conomy reports data on a control group of 11 persons with nontraumatic spinal cord lesions and found that most of the patients denied any disorder of body image. When they did occur, the experience was fragmentary, brief, and nonrecurrent. Paresthesias and pain were reported but no experience of distorted position sense. Conomy concludes by noting that body image distortions may occur more frequently than we believe because physicians may not interview the person to obtain this data, and, perhaps more importantly, the patients may be reluctant to discuss any body image distortions because they fear it indicates psychological disturbance on their part. Although Conomy obtained his data by interview and it should be replicated, he gives excellent descriptions of the body image phenomena experienced by his patients. This article should be consulted by anyone who works with persons with spinal injury or who plans research into this area.

Studies of body image as a personality variable in persons with spinal cord injury have not produced much information that is helpful in understanding the process of adjustment to spinal injury. Wachs and Zaks (1960) administered the Draw-A-Person test to two groups of persons. The spinal injury group consisted of 30 traumatically injured males with an average length of hospitalization of 5.4 years and the control group consisted of 30 male inpatients with "incurable" chronic diseases with an average length of hospitalization of 2.5 months. The groups were comparable on average age and education. There were 60 drawings of the human form by these subjects which were analyzed for abnormality in the drawing. Among the 30 most pathological drawings, there were an equal number by the spinal injury groups and the control group. An analysis of 24 variables within these drawings produced few differences between the two groups.

Dimond and Hirt (1973) were quite interested in body involvement in schizophrenic subjects, so they used persons with paraplegia and a normal control group to make comparisons in response to the Secord Homonym Test as a measure of total body association. Persons with paraplegia showed more "body involvement" than the nondisabled control group and the schizophrenic group; thus they conclude that body image distortions are not prominent in schizophrenics.

Rosillo and Fogel (1971) found almost no relationship between body image and improvement in rehabilitation in their study, but, despite this fact, caution us not to discard the body image variable; they proceed to discuss its importance to rehabilitation.

Landau (1960) found that barrier scores on the Rorschach were positively related to adjustment to physical handicap (defined by scores on a psychosocial rating scale constructed for the study; reliability was established but not validity). Mitchell (1970) studied the relation of barrier scores to adjustment in persons with paraplegia and quadriplegia. There were 50 persons in the former group and 52 persons in the latter group. Each person was categorized as high adjustment or low adjustment according to scores on tests. He found that barrier score did differentiate between high and low adjustment persons with paraplegia but not in quadriplegia. He concluded that the barrier score is a questionable index of adjustment to stress induced by severe disability.

Arnhoff and Mehl (1963) define body image as the visual memory image one has of one's body and believe that in persons with paraplegia accuracy in judging width of shoulders would deteriorate because this is no longer a relevant dimension in coping with the environment. They predicted that persons with paraplegia would be more accurate in judging width of their wheelchair than shoulder width. Their results do, indeed, confirm their hypothesis.

Consequently, based on these studies, it must be concluded that body image as traditionally defined by personality theorists has not been demonstrated to be a critical variable in the process of adjustment to spinal cord injury. However, the problem has been in the definition of and measurement of body image. Yet the changes in perception of body image which Conomy describes seem to be an interesting area for study, and the implications of his data seem obvious. Newly injured persons should be interviewed to assess the presence of body image distortions and then they should be reassured that this is a very frequent experience following spinal injury and that this experience does not imply that they are psychologically unbalanced.

None of these comments should be interpreted to imply that perception of one's body and feelings about the physical changes associated with spinal injury are not important in the adjustment to such injury. On the contrary, persons with spinal injury describe increased efforts to look attractive since the injury in contrast to a lesser concern with personal appearance prior to injury. These persons believe that how they look and the attitudes that they communicate about their body to others is a big factor in their success in coping with the social world following spinal injury (Consumer Conference 1977).

Pain

Pain, according to Harris and associates (1973), is very often the main problem in acute spinal injury and dominates the patient's mind in the first week after injury. Burke (1973) believes that response to a given painful stimulus is variable from individual to individual and that there is an important psychological component to the sensation of pain. In addition, he notes that there are variations in the reported incidence of pain from different rehabilitation centers. Thus, he compared the incidence of pain problems at two different spinal cord injury centers and found that Austin Hospital in Australia reported that 14 percent of the patients had pain and Rancho Los Amigos Hospital in California reported that 45 percent of the patients complained of pain. Burke wondered if these differences related to the psychological management of the patients at the two centers since he believes that psychological reactions to severe disability are the real cause of excessive response to painful stimuli. One major difference between the two centers was the delay between injury and admission to the spinal injury center. Austin Hospital received most of its patients immediately after injury, whereas at Rancho, acute treatment of the injury was given at another hospital for weeks or months before admission to Rancho. Thus, poor medical and psychological management of the person in the early phases seemed to be an important factor in the higher incidence of pain problems at Rancho. An examination of readmissions at Rancho found that many of the readmissions among the pain patients were for pressure sores. Seventy-five percent of the persons in the pain group at Rancho who were readmitted were known or probable drug abusers. More persons with paraplegia were in the pain group than persons with quadriplegia at both centers. One other factor in the different incidence of pain was the greater amount of surgery performed on the Rancho group, most of it before admission to Rancho, however. Thus, scarring was a factor in the pain problems. This study must be commended for its multifaceted evaluation of the problem of pain in spinal injury. Not only are physical factors discussed but the interaction between the physical and psychological reactions to spinal cord injury is emphasized.

Hohmann (1975) states that patients with spinal injury seem to describe four kinds of pain problems. Phantom sensations are frequent in the early stages of injury but are not usually perceived as painful unless this expectancy has been set by the staff or other patients. He advises that the patients should be counseled not to be worried by these experiences. Burning-tingling sensations, of the cord injured, are almost universally described, he states, and are similar to the feeling that the part has "gone to sleep." Training the person to suppress or ignore the sensation is advised and neurosurgical and chemotherapeutic approaches are usually not successful remedies. Radicular pain may be observed early after injury and tends to diminish in a few weeks. Causalgialike pain is almost exclusively described by patients with cauda equina or incomplete lesions and is described as a shooting or electric pain. Hohmann explains that if this experience is described by a person with a lesion above T_{11}, it is associated with either an incomplete lesion, with psychological disturbances, an addiction problem, or the person has learned to interpret his symptoms in this manner after observing another patient do so. Furthermore, this is the only type of pain that responds favorably to neurosurgical intervention, such as spinothalomic tractotomy.

Hohmann advises conservative management of pain problems and, if surgery is considered, a thorough psychological evaluation should be performed to screen out associated psychological difficulties. Mueller (1962b) describes the use of the Rorschach to predict successful relief of pain following chordotomy. On a sample of 14 patients, the Rorschach successfully predicted relief of pain in 10 cases, 2 were "misses," and 2 doubtful. Thus, Mueller strongly concurs with Hohmann in emphasizing the need for examining the psychological components to a pain problem.

Fordyce, Fowler, Lehmann, DeLateur, Sand, and Trieschmann (1973) have pioneered in creating a program of psychological management of pain problems using behavior therapy techniques. This approach has been found to be successful in certain cases where there is no physical treatment available that would successfully eliminate the pain without significant side effects. Although the research has been done on persons with low back pain, the behavioral approach to pain in persons with spinal injury has considerable relevance. To obtain more information on this approach, the book by Fordyce (1976) is recommended.

The role of drugs was mentioned by Burke (1973), who noted a higher incidence of alcohol and drug abuse among the Rancho pain patients. He wonders if those who take drugs and alcohol in large quantities have a lower pain threshold and suggests that this is symptomatic of an inability to cope with stress both before and after the spinal injury. The Vista Hill Psychiatric Foundation (1974) is concerned about the drug-dependent person with paraplegia and notes that iatrogenic factors should not be overlooked. Persons with spinal injury have been very vocal about the large amounts of medication that seemed to be pushed upon them, usually without explanation as to what its purpose was. It also seemed to them that some medical personnel appeared to be overly reliant on dispensing medication as a way to deal with many problems. Often the consumers did not want to take any more pills, but they had no choice.

Dunn and Davis (1974) describe an informal survey of ten patients with spinal injury who admitted to the use of marijuana. Fifty percent of the group report a decrease in spasticity and headache pain after smoking marijuana. The authors suggest that a controlled study be conducted to replicate these findings and that these results should be considered as hypotheses only until confirmed by further research.

Thus, pain is a complex phenomenon that can play an important role in the adjustment to spinal cord injury depending on the person's preinjury style of coping with stress and depending upon the manner in which the rehabilitation staff react to the pain problem. Treatment factors can predispose a person to more pain than necessary (such as excessive surgery or complications associated with poor management of the problem), but the degree and style of the person's reaction will depend on his personality style and the type of attention the environment gives to his pain reaction. Therefore, the behavioral aspects of pain management are very relevant to spinal injury as a prevention of iatrogenic problems and as a treatment approach.

Reactions of Rehabilitation Personnel

The reactions of rehabilitation personnel can be a factor in the psychological adjustment to spinal cord injury. If the staff of a rehabilitation center tend to have certain perceptions of persons with spinal injury, these perceptions form part of the psychological climate of a hospital. In addition, if there are certain generalized perceptions that rehabilitation staff do have about persons with spinal injury, they may influence the outcome of research projects that use ratings by staff as a measure of the criterion variable.

Taylor (1967) studied the immediate reactions of persons with spinal injury and compared these actual reactions to the psychological reactions predicted by experienced and naive subjects. The experienced group were rehabilitation personnel at a prominent rehabilitation center, and the naive group were college fraternity men. The measurement of reaction to spinal injury was on the Minnesota Multiphasic Personality Inventory (MMPI). The experienced and naive groups were asked to fill out the MMPI in a manner that would describe the reactions of a person who had recently received a spinal injury. These data were compared to the actual responses on the MMPI by a group of 47 males with spinal injury.

The persons with spinal injury described themselves on the MMPI as quite similar to the average male university student. There was evidence of only mild depression. However, the data revealed that neither the experienced nor the naive predictors had a clear and accurate idea of the psychological reactions of cord injured patients who were within three months of injury. Both predictor groups displayed a high degree of agreement in the response patterns on the MMPI, the predictions of both groups being consistent with the widely held, stable, and negative stereotype of the disabled person. The average profiles predicted by both groups suggested acute psychic distress, depression, anxiety, bizarre mentation, and somatic overconcern. Item analyses revealed these content clusters: social isolation or withdrawal; alienation from and rejection by society; feelings of hopelessness, depression, and anxiety; lack of self-confidence; marked sensitivity, especially about somatic appearance. These predicted responses were not at all consistent with the perceptions that the persons with spinal cord injury had about themselves.

What is striking about Taylor's study is that the rehabilitation personnel who had worked with many persons with spinal cord injury were no better at predicting the psychological reaction to spinal injury than persons who had had no contact with any disabled persons. Both groups vastly overestimated the degree of psychological distress that a person would (or should?) feel in such a situation.

Klas (1970) used staff ratings of depression as one of the measures of his criterion and found that the staff rated most patients as being more depressed than the patients rated themselves. Albrecht and Higgins (1977) found a low correlation between patients' self-ratings and staff ratings of psychological processes in adjustment to disability. Lawson (1976), who used multiple levels of measurement of depression, concludes that nursing notes or ratings by others are not good indicators of what is going on inside the patient.

As we consider staff reactions and the psychological climate that this creates within a rehabilitation center, the study by Antler, Lee, Zaretsky, Pezenik, and Halberstam (1969) should be noted. They had persons with both severe and mild disabilities rate their attitude toward the wheelchair. This was to be used as a measure of change in value structure of the patients which was hypothesized to correlate with acceptance of the disability. Nondisabled re-habilitation staff members also rated their attitudes toward the wheelchair. These authors found that the mildly disabled persons rated the wheelchair more positively than the more severely disabled persons did, perhaps because the former group needed the wheelchair only temporarily. However, the nondisabled staff rated the wheelchair more negatively than either of the disabled patient groups. The authors conclude that this negative rating by the staff may be related to a negative stereotype of the disabled which is held by the nondisabled. Furthermore, they note that the more disabled person was closer to the nondisabled person in their perception of the wheelchair. "Thus, the severely disabled person may be consonant in his self-image with the stereotype held regarding him by nondisabled persons" (Antler et al. 1969, p. 51).

Taylor (1974) studied the goals that occupational therapists (OT) have for persons with quadriplegia and with paraplegia and compared these goals with the goals that persons with these disabilities had for themselves in OT. She found that persons with quadriplegia identified work tolerance, muscle strengthening, bowel and bladder control, wheelchair mobility and transfer-ring as their most important goals. Occupational therapists rated development of adapted equipment and devices as the most important goal, followed by eating, socialization, wheelchair mobility, and writing/typing. However, persons with quadriplegia ranked development of assistive devices as thirteenth in importance to them. There was a less marked discrepancy between OTs and persons with paraplegia in terms of goals for the treatment. Taylor concluded by noting that,

Therapists may not be communicating with patients what they perceive the goals of treatment to be or they may not be acting upon the feedback from patients regarding their wants and goals. If it is assumed that active patient involvement in treatment is desirable, effective communication between therapists and patients is vital. (D. Taylor 1974, p. 29)

Morgan, Hohmann, and Davis (1974) surveyed the VA spinal cord injury centers and found that staff expectations for patient performance were quite negative. Only 30 percent of the staff members interviewed believed that most persons with spinal injury could ultimately live out in the community. Seventy-one percent of the staff believed that persons with spinal injury were different from others with handicaps, and 60 percent believed that persons with spinal injury were more difficult to motivate to do things for themselves than other persons with handicaps.

Albrecht and Higgins (1977) comment about staff reactions to patients who do not adopt the traditional sick role. They state:

> After extensive observation of staff conferences, it became apparent that medical-rehabilitation staff do not seem prepared to accept these new patient roles and therefore judge some of these independent patients to be uncooperative and not to have completed the staff's conception of the rehabilitation program. (Albrecht and Higgins 1977, p. 44)

These data tend to suggest that many rehabilitation personnel have preconceived ideas about the psychological reaction to spinal injury and the roles that patients should play. They tend to perceive more psychological suffering than persons with spinal injury describe. This bias, then, complicates the interpretation of research in which staff ratings are a measure of the criterion. In addition, this bias may reflect an expectation that the staff have about the expected reaction to spinal injury. This could create a psychological climate in which the person with spinal injury realizes that everyone considers him to be very unfortunate. He senses that he is expected to experience great psychological distress. Lawson (1977), as previously noted, reports that the most depressing experience for his sample was the staff expectation that they should be depressed. This is, indeed, the requirement of mourning that Dembo, Leviton, and Wright (1975) describe. In addition, it appears that we, rehabilitation personnel, impose the same requirement of mourning that the general public does.

Persons with spinal injury are quite concerned by the unrealistic attitudes and ideas that many rehabilitation personnel have. Especially for persons with quadriplegia, rehabilitation staff are very conservative in their ideas as to what may be possible for the person following discharge. There is an unwillingness to allow the person to try a living arrangement that is less than ideal even though the only alternative may be a nursing home or living with parents. Many decisions on physical management and adaptive equipment are made without considering all of the functional implications of that decision. For example, some centers try to eliminate all indwelling catheters before discharge from the hospital in order to prevent bladder infections. Yet the presence or absence of an indwelling catheter for a female with quadriplegia may be the prime factor in her ability to be independent in certain phases of her life. Without the catheter, she must have physical assistance available 24 hours a day for toileting activities. But with the catheter, she can have greater freedom and more opportunities for home, social, vocational, and recreational activities. Furthermore, many rehabilitation therapists never ask the person with the disability what his or her goals are for the therapy (Consumer Conference 1977).

Our belief that the person is, indeed, unfortunate, may be communicated, subtly, by our attitudes toward the wheelchair and our emphasis on braces and splints, whereas research shows that the person often discards these devices after discharge (Grynbaum, Kaplan, Lloyd, and Rusk 1963). Professionals talk about the importance of having the patient participate in the goal-setting and decision-making process, but is the person with spinal injury actually consulted? And what if his goals or decisions are not the same as the team's? Whose decisions prevail? Professionals state that the goals for the person are independence to the degree that he or she is capable, but he is rated as uncooperative if he asserts his independence in determining how his time will be used in the rehabilitation center. Thus, the psychological climate in a rehabilitation center may be one that shapes a perception of oneself as less competent than before the injury. This is an area that must be explored as a policy and research issue for the future.

How do staff behaviors toward patients influence the course of rehabilitation? How do patients feel about staff behavior toward them and does this affect the process of adjustment to spinal cord injury? How much of the adaptive equipment prescribed is actually used by the person after discharge? What are the functional implications for independence of many of the decisions labeled as medical management? Why do professionals constantly refer to disabled people as patients even after they are no longer in the hospital? What is the effect of language on the image of the person with a disability? What is communicated by calling somebody a "para" or a "quad" rather than a person with paraplegia or a person with quadriplegia? Consequently, one must ask what procedures can be implemented that permit the person with a disability to participate in the decision-making process and to take steps to manage his or her own life?

PERSONALITY CHARACTERISTICS OF PERSONS WITH SPINAL CORD INJURY

Is there a spinal cord injury personality? Professionals concur that there is no unitary personality style associated with any disability (Wright 1960; Siller 1969; Shontz 1971; Cook 1976). However, there have been a few efforts to determine if there are some preinjury personality characteristics that persons with spinal cord injury share.

Fordyce (1964) studied a sample of males with spinal injury who had been categorized into two groups: those whose disability occurred as a result of their own imprudent behavior and those whose injury occurred through accident with no evidence of imprudence on their parts. He found that the group categorized as imprudent onset scored higher on scales 3 and 4 of the Minnesota Multiphasic Personality Inventory (MMPI) than the prudent group. These scores generally reflect a tendency toward impulse-dominated behavior, some aggressiveness, and some poor judgment.

In a related study, Kunce and Worley (1966) tested two groups on the Strong Vocational Interest Blank (SVIB). One group was composed of those who were active agents in their accidents, and the other group consisted of those who were passive agents. Those who were active agents in their accidents scored higher on the aviator key of the SVIB, which is often interpreted as showing evidence of adventurousness, boldness, and assertiveness.

Since we know that 82 percent of spinal injuries occur in males, most of whom are young and active, these results may reflect the influence of age and sex variables. Fordyce (1964) does report that those in his imprudent group tended to be younger than those in his prudent group. Dinsdale, Lesser, and Judd (1971) think that persons with spinal injury might be categorized into three groups: young, unmarried males; married, somewhat older males; and married females. They believe that the younger, unmarried males exhibit the most problems.

However, Bourestom and Howard (1965) and Taylor (1967) found that the average MMPI profiles of persons with spinal injury reflected only mild depression with only slight elevations on scales related to impulsivity and energy level. Taylor described the average MMPI profile of his group as similar to that of male university students. Therefore, we should be aware of the base rate for high energy and impulsivity in the age group 15–25, which is the age group during which a large proportion of spinal injuries occur.

The averaging of MMPI profiles for a heterogeneous group may lead to assumptions or interpretations that really do not characterize many members of the group. This issue will be discussed in a later section. Therefore, the approach of Fordyce and Kunce and Worley may be more appropriate: categorize people on the basis of their actual behavior and then determine if there are any ways in which the groups differ. Their information is very interesting and, with careful consideration of the base rates, their results should be considered to be hypotheses for future research. Cook (1976) suggests that a substantial proportion of persons who receive spinal injuries were experiencing psychological disruption prior to injury. Hohmann (1975) believes that a significant proportion of the spinal injury population may have preexisting personality problems. However, at this time we have no data to substantiate these notions; therefore, careful research is necessary.

If one were to divide all activities into three broad categories, the categories might be labeled: motor-physical, verbal-intellectual, and social-interpersonal. Many activities might fit into two categories, and some activities might be difficult to label (for example, is playing the flute strictly a motor activity?). All people have activities in each category, but some people may have a large proportion of their activities in one category versus another. Those people whose work and leisure activities are in the motor-physical area might find the onset of spinal injury to have a greater impact on their lives than a person whose activities are in the verbal-intellectual area. Locus of control may play a big role in how one manages after spinal injury, but the amount of behavioral change required might be reflected by these categories of activities.

The manner in which a person handled anger and frustration may influence reaction to disability. Those whose anger was dissipated through motor activity may find that spinal injury has eliminated or restricted this avenue of control. Thus, increased physical activity within the limits of the disability may be very helpful to this group.

Within the group who receive a spinal injury, very few display gross evidence of psychopathology following the onset (Nagler 1950; Munro 1954). Some transient states of psychological disorganization may occur, but usually these are related to sensory deprivation factors. Hohmann (1975) believes that if the person has a preinjury history of severe depression, especially if it resulted in hospitalization or suicide attempts, the prognosis for adjustment to spinal injury will be poor. In a similar fashion, any evidence of preinjury inability to cope with stress over a significant period of time does not appear to portend well for coping with a disability. Psychiatric hospitalizations, suicide attempts, and severe alcohol and drug abuse may be signs of inability to handle stress prior to injury.

Yet Hohmann (1975) reports that in a study of 18 men with spinal injury who were overtly psychotic at the time of injury, the overt psychotic symptomatology disappeared within a few days of injury although the secondary symptoms of psychosis remained (flat affect, thought disorder). Furthermore, the overt psychotic symptoms did not recur unless the lesion was incomplete and there was a return of function, or until the person was pressured to leave the sheltered environment of the hospital. These persons responded fairly well to the usual rehabilitation program, and they seemed to need fewer drugs for their psychological state than the nondisabled schizophrenic psychiatric population.

Vash (1975) is concerned that looking for preexisting personality disorders will obscure the need to pay attention to the tremendous psychological impact that disability may have because of reality problems in the patient's social world. She is concerned that rehabilitation staff use psychological tests to categorize people rather than to devote the time to listening to them and helping them to resolve the reality problems they face.

Thus, we have little data on the personality characteristics of the population with spinal injury. There is enough evidence in the literature to indicate that this group is a heterogeneous one. Consequently, it may be more profitable to discard our efforts to describe typical groups and instead collect behavioral data in an empirical manner, and, after many years, sort the data and see how they fall.

Persons with traumatically induced spinal cord injury comprise a heterogeneous population when they arrive for treatment: age, sex, cultural structure, education, marital status, experience in working and living, are as divergent as human nature itself. They will continue to be a heterogeneous group when they leave the centers, with one obvious difference: they will demonstrate a severe and probably permanent physical impairment. (Wilcox and Stauffer 1972, p. 115)

This caution seems to be appropriate when attempts are made to identify personality characteristics associated with spinal injury or factors associated with adjustment to disability.

FACTORS ASSOCIATED WITH ADJUSTMENT TO SPINAL CORD INJURY

There have been a fair number of studies that have attempted to identify those characteristics that are associated with successful adjustment to spinal cord injury. Unfortunately, these studies rarely define adjustment in a similar manner; thus, it is difficult to compare the results.

Nickerson (1971) studied 48 persons with spinal cord injury who were rated as to their hospital adjustment, which was defined as normality of function within the limitation set by the person's handicap. The criterion for hospital adjustment was the degree to which the person had met and cooperated with the hospital rehabilitation objective set for him. Criteria for out of hospital adjustment were the establishment of feasible vocational and housing plans as well as maintenance of affectional or family ties. A number of psychological tests were administered to these persons and correlated with the ratings of adjustment.

Nickerson found that adjustment to paraplegia was significantly related to educational and occupational attainment and to theoretical vocational interests. These factors also correlated with socioeconomic level. In addition, she found that financial resources were important to adjustment to the handicap.

This study has some methodological problems that make generalization of the results difficult. We have no information about the subject population in this study, e.g., severity of injury, duration of disability, and age. Adjustment was defined as cooperation with hospital procedures which in Kalb's (1971) study was shown to correlate negatively with the range of behaviors outside of the hospital. In addition, adjustment outside of the hospital was rated on the basis of behaviors occurring while in the hospital. Thus, at best we can conclude that education and theoretical interests, in this study, correlated with cooperation with hospital procedures in this group.

Kemp and Vash (1971) carried out an excellent study which could be a model for the cross-sectional type of research into the outcomes of spinal injury. They selected 50 persons with spinal injury who had been injured at least 5 years with an average duration of 11 years. There were 25 persons with paraplegia and 25 with quadriplegia, and the distribution by sexes was similar to that in the hospital population of persons with spinal injury; 18 in each group were males. They were interviewed for an average of 2.5 hours using a structured interview, and a series of psychological tests were administered. Based on data from the interviews, independent judges rated the productivity of the persons based on data regarding vocational, educational, leisure, home, and group membership information. They tested the following independent variables: level of injury, sex, age at onset, age now, duration of disability, material resources, years employed preinjury, educational level preinjury, information subscale score, goals now, interpersonal support received now, greatest loss now. These variables were correlated with the productivity ratings using multiple regression analyses.

They found that the factors contributing most to the prediction of productivity were number of reported goals, the reported greatest loss, a creativity test (Seeing Problems), and age now. Number of reported goals contributed most to the prediction of productivity, accounting for almost 50 percent of the total variance. There was a significant interaction between age and goals. Younger persons with many goals were more productive than older persons reporting many goals.

Interpersonal support and level of injury produced a significant interaction. With high support, there were no differences by level of injury. With less support, persons with paraplegia were significantly more productive than persons with quadriplegia. The goals expressed by less productive persons were primarily materialistic, avocational, and physical functioning goals. The more productive persons expressed goals in vocational, materialistic, and family-interpersonal areas. The groups were equal on materialistic goals only. In addition, productive persons expressed significantly more new goals than less productive persons, regardless of level of injury or duration of disability.

Productive persons scored high on scales of dominance, social presence, and self-acceptance on the California Psychological Inventory. Less productive persons were at least one standard deviation below the mean of the nondisabled population on many scales. On tests of creativity, the most productive persons scored significantly higher than less productive persons and general psychology students. However, there was no relationship between productivity and preinjury type of employment.

This study is an example of the kind of quality research that can be conducted if the investigators give attention to the number of variables that can influence the results. With more research of this caliber, the state of the art would advance rapidly.

Kalb (1971) studied the relationship between depression and noncooperation in the hospital and postdischarge behaviors. This study was reviewed in detail in the section on depression but will be briefly noted again. For middle-class persons, noncooperation on the ward was positively correlated with the range of postdischarge behaviors. Depression in these subjects was unrelated to behavior after discharge. But for lower-class subjects, depression correlated negatively with all 11 outcome variables. Ward noncooperation did not correlate with postdischarge behavior, except involvement in school and employment which showed a negative correlation. Low SES subjects who were noncooperative during hospitalization tended to have preinjury histories of trouble adjusting to society. This was not the case for the middle SES subjects.

Kerr and Thompson (1972) followed 181 persons with spinal injury and rated their mental adjustment to the disability as failure, poor, fair, good, and excellent. Unfortunately, the methodology for obtaining these rates was not specified. They found that the young tended to adjust better than the old (over 45 years). But whether this was age at follow-up or age at onset was unspecified. In addition, 53 percent of those rated as having failed in mental adjustment had unsatisfactory preinjury life histories, whereas 29 percent had satisfactory preinjury life histories. Of those rated as having made an excellent adjustment, all had satisfactory preinjury life histories.

For the entire group of 181 persons with spinal injuries, their rated adjustments by category were: failure, 9 percent; poor, 13 percent; fair, 22 percent; good, 39 percent; excellent, 17 percent. All of those rated as having made an excellent adjustment came from exceptionally warm and loving backgrounds. Eight of the 11 failures in the over age 45 category were dead at follow-up, and 7 of these 8 had unsatisfactory previous life histories or had severe unresolved problems before onset of the disability.

Level of lesion was unrelated to successful adjustment. Those who returned to the hospital repeatedly with medical problems and pressure sores tended to have significant unresolved psychological problems (unspecified). Of the 30 persons rated as having an excellent adjustment, only one had financial difficulties; thus, Kerr and Thompson are convinced that financial security is a major factor in adjustment.

This study provides some interesting data which can be used as hypotheses for future research. Unfortunately, what criteria they used to rate adjustment to disability or satisfactory versus unsatisfactory preinjury history is not known. Therefore, it is not known if their figure indicating that 56 percent make excellent or good adjustments is representative of the general population of spinal injury. Also, one would wonder if the 44 percent rated as failure, poor, or fair were predetermined to be in these categories because of their age and previous life history, or whether intensive psychosocial rehabilitation would improve the success rate. This question becomes a critical one and perhaps is the key question in regard to outcome.

Wilcox and Stauffer (1972) noted that older persons at injury seemed to be least affected by vocational and social rehabilitation efforts. Although they learned some self-care, they needed help from family and attendants and demonstrated the least progress at follow-up. The youngest group seemed to be the most malleable and responsive to all types of rehabilitation efforts and appeared to adapt to a complicated new way of life, despite the particularly large number of cervical injuries among them.

Athelstan and Crewe (1978) conducted a follow-up study of 126 persons with spinal injury using a questionnaire and a lengthy interview. These persons were categorized according to the circumstances of their accident as innocent victims, passively involved, or actively involved. The latter group were involved in accidents resulting from obvious negligence, poor judgment, or voluntarily entering into a high risk situation. Interestingly, in the innocent victim category, persons with quadriplegia accounted for only 17 percent of the group. All persons in the sample were rated on psychosocial, vocational, and medical adjustment without knowledge of type of accident.

Contrary to clinical lore, the group of innocent victims received consistently poorer ratings of adjustment than the other two groups, and those who were actively involved in their accident received the most favorable ratings in each area of adjustment. Forty-four percent of the actively involved group were employed full time in comparison to 28 percent of the innocent victims. Innocent victims reported much less constructive activity and more hospitalizations than the other groups.

The authors, surprised by their results, conclude that, ''the foolish risk takers may also be energetic, adventuresome, and adaptable [and] these characteristics may be the ones which most influence long term adjustment, despite early difficulties'' (Athelstan and Crewe 1979, p. 10).

Carlson (1974) followed up a sample of 54 persons with spinal injury and found that in general they were quite satisfied with life but dissatisfaction occurred most frequently in family and other interpersonal relationships. Those who scored higher on conceptual abstractness tended to be somewhat more satisfied with life, and there was a correlation between the ability to articulate goals and satisfaction with life.

In summary, these studies suggest that youth, financial security, warm, loving backgrounds, and interpersonal support are important variables which favor good adjustment to disability. Such intrapersonal characteristics as a certain amount of independence and aggressiveness, intellectual interests, creativity, and having many goals may also be associated with good adjustment to spinal injury. However, many of the studies used different definitions of adjustment, often not clearly specified, and Albrecht and Higgins (1977) demonstrate the importance of this concept. They found that many different measures of outcome or success in a rehabilitation program correlated poorly. Improvement in physical function correlated little with staff ratings of psychological adjustment in the patients. In addition, there was little correlation between staff ratings of adjustment to disability and the patients' self-ratings.

THE CORRELATION OF PERSONALITY CHARACTERISTICS AND DECUBITUS ULCER INCIDENCE

Anderson and Andberg (1977) did a follow-up study of persons with spinal injury to assess the number of days lost because of pressure sores and found that the persons with paraplegia had a significantly greater number of days interrupted by pressure sores and spent more days hospitalized for pressure sores than persons with quadriplegia. Comparing each of these two groups according to degree of responsibility for skin care produced some interesting results. Persons with paraplegia who had help with skin care reported the most number of days interrupted by pressure sores, whereas the persons with quadriplegia who were independent in skin care had the best record. When the sample was divided into two groups according to days interrupted by pressure sores, high and low, and compared on psychosocial variables, the group with no days lost from pressure sores scored higher on responsibility, both in practice and in attitude toward maintaining the integrity of their skin. Also, they scored significantly higher on the amount of satisfaction they obtained from their activities of life than those with more days lost from pressure sores. Scores on a test of self-esteem were not significantly different for the two groups.

Furthermore, dividing the groups into level of injury revealed that persons with paraplegia who had help with skin care reported significantly less personal responsibility in skin care when compared to persons with paraplegia and quadriplegia who were independent in skin care. These persons tended to view skin breakdown as an event which was caused by something outside of their responsibility. Self-esteem did not correlate with days lost because of pressure sores, but those who reported a greater amount of satisfaction with activities of life had a higher self-esteem. Using a regression analysis, the variables that accounted for a greater amount of variance in the number of days lost because of pressure sores was satisfaction with activities of life.

Using an empirical and promising approach, Brockway (1978) studied the base rate of decubitus ulcer incidence for persons with spinal injury at one of the regional spinal injury centers and then attempted to determine if persons with certain personality types were likely to acquire decubitus ulcers more frequently than the average frequency of occurrence (base rate) of this skin problem. By use of the MMPI, she discovered that persons with a 6–8 profile had a significantly higher incidence of decubitus ulcers than the base rate. No other profile type exceeded the base rate. These data are fascinating since persons with 6–8 MMPI profiles tend to feel a sense of alienation from society and their peer groups and tend to view forces outside of their own control as having a powerful impact on what happens to them. They may not feel the same sense of responsibility for their body nor care about their body and what happens to it. Consequently, it would be interesting to know how such individuals would score on the locus of control dimension.

Thus, acceptance of responsibility for one's body has been viewed as prerequisite for adaptation to the physical changes spinal injury entails. These two studies provide evidence that this seems to be the case in regard to decubitus ulcer incidence. Consequently, more research in this area is needed. These data, however, point up the necessity of planning rehabilitation programs that do indeed teach people to accept responsibility for their own bodies while they are in the hospital and to have these habits well established prior to discharge from the rehabilitation center. Thus, it is proposed that the learning model would be more effective than the medical model as a means of preventing decubitus ulcers. This issue should be tested.

PSYCHOLOGICAL TESTS AND SPINAL CORD INJURY

Psychologists tend to use psychological tests to evaluate persons, and, therefore, the results of studies using these instruments with persons with spinal injury should be examined. Manson (1950) administered the California Test of Mental Maturity, Advanced '47 S-Form; the Otis Quick-Scoring Mental Ability Test, Gamma Form Am; and the Wechsler-Bellevue Scale Form I. He found that a group of 102 males with paraplegia obtained a mean IQ in the average range and concluded that the onset of spinal injury did not lead to mental deterioration due to the injuries.

Hirschenfang and Benton (1966) administered the Rorschach to five persons with quadriplegia and five with paraplegia. They report that the average number of responses for persons with paraplegia is greater than for persons with quadriplegia, but they perform no statistical analyses to assess the significance of this reported difference. The range of responses for the former group is 8–18 and for the latter group, 8–11. Thus, for the ten Rorschach cards, their data base for this study is one or occasionally two responses per card for persons with paraplegia and usually one response per card for persons with quadriplegia. The authors give no information on duration of disability but the average age was 42–43, average education was ninth grade, and the average IQ was 88–93. They interpret the Rorschach results as suggesting that persons with paraplegia manifest childlike, immediate needs for gratification together with difficulties in interpersonal relationships. They claim that persons with quadriplegia appear to be more absorbed with the disability and show a great deal of concern about the human body.

The MMPI has been used in several studies and the results must be examined carefully. Bourestom and Howard (1965) studied three disability groups, arthritis, multiple sclerosis, and spinal cord injury and obtained average MMPI profiles. They found that the group with spinal injury tended to be less depressed and distressed on the average than the other two groups. There were differences in average profiles when males were compared to females in all three groups.

Flynn and Salomone (1977) used the MMPI to predict rehabilitation outcome of 64 clients who were considered to be successful and 64 nonsuccessful at a vocational rehabilitation center. The subjects were severely disabled but type of disability was unspecified. They found that the MMPI was not a good predictor of outcome in multidisabled clients and proposed that measures of actual behavior on the job are a better predictor of vocational success.

Taylor (1967, 1970) used the MMPI with a group of males with spinal injury. Part of this study was described in an earlier section on staff reaction to disability. However, in addition to those results, he found that there are 12 items that persons with spinal cord injury tend to answer in the "pathological" direction but which are merely accurate descriptions of their actual physical condition, such as, "I have difficulty starting and holding my urine." These items are scored on several of the MMPI scales, and elimination of these items significantly changes the shape of and reduces the elevation of the profile. Kendall, Edinger, and Eberly (1978) have confirmed this effect. Thus, Taylor's study suggests that the profiles of persons with spinal injury are artificially elevated because of an artifact in the test situation; we should use caution in interpreting any profile that does not correct for this.

In this regard, the Bourestom and Howard (1965) data represent uncorrected profiles on persons with spinal injury. We would have to conclude, therefore, that the differences they report among the three disability groups are conservative estimates, and the persons with spinal injury may be even less distressed than they report. However, one might speculate that if there are 12 items that artificially inflate the scores of persons with spinal injury, there may be some items that produce this effect in other disability groups. Consequently, this issue should be the focus of research, and all clinicians should read Taylor's study (1970) and correct the profiles of persons with spinal injury accordingly.

Yet one must ask, again, why we would anticipate a homogeneous personality reaction to spinal cord injury when the one feature these persons have in common is the physical disability. This homogeneity of response is an implicit assumption whenever one considers average MMPI profiles or average scores on other measures. Trieschmann and Sand (1971), using terminal renal patients, studied the intellectual and personality response to the process of renal failure. The average MMPI was similar in shape to those in the Bourestom and Howard (1965) study, and the average profiles showed a very low correlation to measures of kidney function. However, when the MMPIs were sorted according to types of responses to the crisis situation, five different reaction types seemed to occur. It was hypothesized that a person's response to impending death would be similar to one's typical response to severe stress and that people differ in these response styles. Thus, five different average profiles were obtained, none of which were similar to the total group average profile. There were vast individual differences which were obscured by the averaging process, and the total average profile was not very descriptive of anyone in the study sample. As a result, this challenges the concept of averaging MMPI profiles or other tests of personality for heterogeneous groups of people. One wonders if sorting the MMPI profiles of persons with spinal injury would lead to the identification of several different reaction types to spinal injury. Does the reaction to disability on the MMPI vary according to age or duration of disability? Is there a difference between males and females? All of these questions should be investigated.

Therefore, descriptions of the average person with spinal injury based on psychological test data should be made with great caution. However, there is little evidence in the literature to indicate that the usual and currently used psychological tests measure variables that are most relevant to functional performance in life following spinal injury. Measures of locus of control show some promise of relating to behaviors relevant to the outcomes of rehabilitation programs. But few other psychological instruments do. It is recommended, therefore, that researchers place more emphasis on direct measures of behavior and use multiple measures of the behavior in question. Clinicians should use direct behavioral observation and interview, in addition to psychological test data, in order to assess an individual with spinal injury.

SUMMARY

The literature reviewed in this section varies in quality. Some of the research has been very good, some very bad. Many articles have been written describing the reaction to spinal cord injury based on the author's own observations or opinion. But there has not been a great deal of research to substantiate these opinions.

The very early stages of spinal injury have not been studied in terms of psychological reaction. Probably most PSV personnel are not on the scene during the acute stage, but any opinions expressed in the literature tend to describe a state of psychological shock characterized by denial of the disability. There is no evidence at this time to demonstrate that this is the case. The position taken in this document is that such descriptions of psychological shock and denial may be an overinterpretation of the situation. Rather, pain, fear about survival, sensory and perceptual deprivation, sleep disruption, and drugs may account for a large part of the person's behavior during this period. This is not to say that the person is not worried, scared, and very upset. But this distress may not be a function of the implications of the disability per se but may relate to these other immediate aversive aspects of the procedures required to insure survival itself.

When survival has been assured, relatively, the person has time to begin to focus on his predicament. The literature contains a great deal of opinion on this issue and, usually, the stages of adjustment are described. These stages are denial, followed by depression; the theory states that depression is necessary for later adjustment to spinal injury. However, there is no research demonstrating that these stages of adjustment do occur, and, in fact, the research suggests that depression may be associated with a less successful adjustment to spinal injury. These results are tentative, and the definition of depression must be agreed upon before these results can be viewed with confidence.

The requirement of mourning has been defined as the belief of nondisabled persons that persons with a disability should mourn their misfortune. This report questions whether some of the descriptions in the literature of the reaction to disability reflect this requirement of mourning rather than the actual reactions to disability. Many studies show that rehabilitation staff consistently overestimate the degree of psychological distress present following disability. Therefore, staff ratings of psychological processes in research studies become suspect. In addition, it is time to declare a moritorium on opinion and emphasize results of good quality research.

Many articles discuss the importance of motivation to the rehabilitation process. Motivation is perceived to be a characteristic within the person which he brings with him to the rehabilitation program. However, using the traditional psychodynamic approach, it is difficult to remedy this motivational deficit through traditional psychological therapies, such as psychotherapy. Therefore, the emphasis has been on the identification of those who have motivation and the attempt to screen out those who do not have motivation. What happens to those who do not have motivation is never specified.

The strict behaviorist believes that motivation is external to the person and consists of those rewards for which the person will work. Remedy for a motivational deficit consists of arranging environmental contingencies to reward the desired behavior. But Seligman describes the state of learned helplessness as the belief that there is no contingency between one's behavior and environmental reward. Rotter's concept of locus of control allows one to predict that those with external locus of control are more susceptible to depression following spinal injury and Seligman sees a relationship between learned helplessness and depression. This may be a very promising area for research in the future. Locus of control and learned helplessness may be very relevant to the concept of motivation, and research into this area may lead to great advances in the treatment of persons with spinal injury. With this approach, no one is screened out, but rather treatment strategies are designed to assist everyone who faces life with a spinal injury.

Body image as a traditionally defined personality construct has not been demonstrated to be relevant to the adjustment to spinal cord injury given the quality of the research up to this time. However, when defined as the interpretation of sensations from various parts of the body, this concept seems to be relevant to spinal injury. It is possible that most newly injured persons with spinal cord lesions experience body image distortions, but there is no evidence as to whether this influences later adjustment to the disability.

Pain behavior is a frequent corollary of spinal injury, and the manner in which it is managed can be very important to later adjustment. Some persons who turn to drugs or alcohol at times of stress may choose this option in the presence of pain. The question remains, however, whether these persons have a lower pain threshold in the beginning. This area is an important one for research. However, the behavioral approach to management of pain may be helpful in cases of pain following spinal injury.

Studies of outcome or adjustment to spinal injury suggest that youth, a good background, interpersonal support, and financial security are important. Some independence and aggressiveness, creativity, many goals for the future all favor good adjustment or productivity after spinal injury. Education and theoretical interests favor vocational success. Basically, it seems that those who were successful at coping with life prior to injury have a greater probability of coping with spinal injury.

As with the concept of motivation, the studies tend to search for intrapersonal or demographic factors that predict successful versus unsuccessful adjustment to spinal injury. If we take data from Kerr and Thompson (1972), 56 percent were rated as good or excellent in adjusting to spinal injury. But what happens to the 44 percent who do not come into the injury situation with these "good" features? The literature does not deal with these persons. Much of our efforts in the literature have been aimed at the identification of variables so that we can predict or "screen out" those who do not have the ability to succeed (do it themselves, essentially). But this is no longer a satisfactory approach given the numbers of persons involved (possibly as many as 44 percent), the costs of repeated medical complications, and the psychosocial stagnation that may occur. Clearly, then, a research goal must be the development of treatment strategies that will give each person the opportunity to live a functional and potentially satisfying life. Thus, it is predicted that such an approach would reduce the costs of spinal cord injury to the nation in the long run, in comparison to our current approach of trying to predict the "winners."

4
Social Factors in the Adjustment to Spinal Cord Injury

Rehabilitation efforts have traditionally focused on teaching the person with spinal cord injury the ADL and mobility techniques that he or she needs to cope with the world. In fact, most measures of success in rehabilitation centers focus on physical skills, and a discharge date is defined in terms of mastering these tasks (Albrecht and Higgins 1977). But are physical skills the appropriate criteria of success in rehabilitation? Does the ability to transfer in and out of a wheelchair or to groom oneself ensure success in coping with the world as a disabled person? The ability to walk and to groom oneself do not ensure success in the world for an able-bodied person since these are tasks that are mastered at ages 5–7 in most persons. After mastery of these physical tasks, life consists of learning to interact with people and the environment in order to get some degree of satisfaction. Thus, the successful able-bodied adult is defined as one who accepts himself and is able to interact with his world to achieve a certain portion of his dreams. Consequently, the same criteria are appropriate for persons with disabilities.

But the onset of a disability, such as spinal cord injury, has tremendous social implications for the disabled person (Safilios-Rothschild 1970). He perceives himself as different, and this is repeatedly confirmed by others' reaction to him. Thus, to cope with the world, he needs to learn a variety of social skills in order to combat the devaluation and rejection he will experience from others. However, the social and ethnic background from which the person comes and to which he will return has an important influence on outcome, as does the impact of the disability on the family. Thus, this chapter will attempt to describe the multitude of social issues that influence the disabled person's attempt to compete in a world designed for and dominated by able-bodied people.

THE SOCIAL IMPLICATIONS OF DISABILITY

Caywood (1974) has described his reaction to the onset of quadriplegia in a most eloquent manner. Very soon after his injury, he realized that people around him displayed pity, sadness, confusion, guilt, and curiosity, and he learned to watch for facial expressions in order to anticipate people's reaction to him. In fact, within a couple of weeks after the injury, he knew that it was his responsibility to put people at ease, and he believes that this becomes a critical skill in the ultimate adjustment to disability.

Several months after his injury when he finally was able to get out of bed, he was shocked to realize how much his body had changed. When he saw himself in a mirror, he did not recognize himself; he had lost 50 pounds, and his clothes were too big for him. Before the accident he had been very strong, but in therapy the task of lifting five pounds seemed like an insurmountable challenge. Thus, the person he had once been was no longer present. He saw himself as very different, and he knew that others also saw the difference.

Toward the end of his inpatient rehabilitation, he was afraid to go home. At the rehabilitation center, he was surrounded by people in the same predicament as his which was comforting; furthermore, the staff members were paid to assist him. As he approached his discharge, he was afraid to be a burden to his family and he felt guilty about disrupting their lives. Indeed, after discharge, it became apparent that the entire family's schedule did revolve around him. But this worry about his family decreased over time since they seemed more than willing to help him. The real shock came when he discovered that the home he remembered fondly was now a house filled with obstacles.

As a quadriplegic, he was not able to go anywhere without assistance from his family, and this was a frustration. Yet at the same time, he did not want to go out into the public world again. He describes himself as an introvert, especially in large groups of people, prior to his accident, but, in addition, he was now self-conscious about being in a wheelchair. His biggest problem in resocialization was the conflict between what he was now—disabled—and how society is structured.

> Society demands that people act and be "normal," not deviate. At the same time, I was constantly reminded that I was not "normal," through interpersonal relationships, architectural barriers, and vocational goals. (Caywood 1974, p. 25)

Thus, Caywood outlined some of the social changes that occurred in his life because of his physical limitations and because of people's reaction to his disability. As a result, social isolation is a very frequent and, unfortunately, a natural feature of postdischarge life unless the person actively fights against it.

To assess the issue of social discomfort following onset of a disability, Dunn (1977) developed a 20-item social discomfort scale and asked persons (males at a veterans hospital) with spinal injury to rate the degree of awkwardness they would feel in various situations. In order of importance, the situations that produce the most discomfort are:

1. Having an accidental bowel movement.
2. Being at a party and discovering that the external catheter has popped.
3. Falling out of the wheelchair.
4. Dealing with people who do not move out of the way.
5. Putting the wheelchair in the car and dealing with a passerby who insists on helping.
6. Being at a bar when a drunk comes up and starts telling you how brave you are.
7. Having spasms in public.
8. Getting on an elevator and having a young girl pat you on the head and say, "Poor dear."
9. Going into a restaurant and the waiter asks your wife or date, "How many please?"

It is interesting to note that Dunn found that men older than age 35 usually admit to more difficulty in these situations than younger men do. One wonders what list of social discomforts would be generated by women with spinal injury.

Cogswell (1968) studied a group of 35 persons with paraplegia who had been out of the rehabilitation center for quite a while (time unspecified). She found that in comparison to pretrauma life, all of the persons with paraplegia, upon returning home, had a marked reduction in: (1) number of social contacts with others in the community; (2) frequency in entering community settings; and (3) number of roles that they played. All of the persons in her study eventually showed an increase in these three activities, but there was tremendous variability in the extent of the increase.

Cogswell and Dunn confirm some of Caywood's observations about the process of adjustment to spinal injury, and their data suggest that there is a considerable degree of agreement as to the social implications of a disability. The concept of self undergoes a change as one learns that people respond differently now that one is disabled. But more importantly, Goffman (1963) believes that the self-concept changes because upon becoming disabled, a person perceives himself with the same degree of negativism as he has viewed others with disabilities or stigmas prior to the injury.

> The painfulness, then, of sudden stigmatization can come not from the individual's confusion about his identity, but from his knowing too well what he has become. (Goffman 1963, p. 133)

Goffman believes that shame becomes an issue in learning to live with a disability and overcoming this shame becomes central to the acceptance of oneself.

Human beings readily categorize each other and develop a set of expectations as to how to react to persons in various categories. But when a person is encountered who does not fit these categories, our expectations become disrupted and we become uneasy in our interactions with the person. This tendency to categorize people and to develop expectations regarding them develops at an early age and becomes a central feature of all interpersonal relationships.

Jones and Sisk (1970) presented 230 children between the ages of 2 and 6 with pictures of orthopedically disabled children and nondisabled children and asked a series of questions designed to elicit their reactions to the pictures. Children aged 2 and 3 did not refer to any disabling feature that differentiated the pictures. However, by age 4, the children were referring to the braces on the legs in the pictures. At age 5, the children spontaneously referred to the children in the pictures as crippled. Thus, as age increased, there was greater accuracy in describing the pictures, and the incidence of perception of disability increased. By age 4, the children were already aware of the functional limitations imposed by an orthopedic disability and had begun to expect different behaviors from those with disabilities.

Richardson (1971) demonstrated that children, aged 10–11, tend to prefer a nonhandicapped white child, a nonhandicapped black child, a facial disfigurement, use of a wheelchair, crutches and leg braces, obesity, and amputation in this order. In another study, Richardson and his colleagues (1961) found that handicapped *and* nonhandicapped children of many cultures rank nonhandicapped children as the preferred companions. Furthermore, they found that disability is a more important element in establishing preference than skin color (Richardson and Royce 1968).

Consequently, it would seem that at an early age we all learn to perceive the differences among people, to form categories, and to place a different valuation on these categories. We prefer some people as companions and reject others. Children learn to reject persons with disabilities although most of them have had little or no contact with disabled children. Thus, the concept of difference is learned along with the tendency to reject those who are different and this seems to be a consistent factor in all prejudice. Friedson (1965) notes that to be handicapped is to be perceived as having an undesirable difference from other people. This early learning of the concept of difference and the rejection of that which is different is reinforced by literature, particularly children's stories which are peopled with ugly witches, hunchbacked gnomes, one-legged evil pirates, and deformed beggars (Reynales 1976). Advertisements and commercials exalt the glories of youth and beauty and suggest that the beautiful people are the most successful and most happy. Products are promoted with the subtle insinuation that use of the product will increase one's attractiveness. Therefore, physical attractiveness and one's perception of one's body do indeed become important aspects of self-concept in adulthood.

Robertiello (1976) believes that there is a double standard in the importance of physical attractiveness between males and females. Men are judged to be desirable because of their personality, intelligence, or success. However, a woman's value is very much judged to be on the basis of her physical attractiveness. Other qualities do not seem to be able to make up for the lack of it.

Berscheid and Walster (1974) tend to agree, but their research shows that physical attractiveness is of major significance for both sexes in dating choice. However, males report that they place more emphasis on physical attractiveness in choosing a partner than women seem to do. These authors review a large amount of research that suggests that physically attractive persons are perceived more favorably along many dimensions than unattractive persons and that this perception is present among children as early as nursery school age. By age 8–10, children rate a pretty face as a primary feature of femaleness and a tall, muscular physique as a criterion for maleness.

If the rejection of differences, disability in particular, and preference for physical attractiveness is learned at an early age and persists into adulthood, then persons who suffer a spinal cord injury have also learned these preferences. Thus, one factor in determining the impact of spinal cord injury may be the emphasis that the person had previously placed on physical attractiveness or prowess as an issue in interacting with the world. Do very attractive persons have a more difficult time adjusting to spinal injury or does the self-confidence they had previously developed assist them in facing social situations? This becomes an interesting issue for research.

If the person with spinal injury has learned to prefer physically attractive people prior to injury, his or her self-concept will be challenged by the onset of the disability. He or she may be very rejecting of this new image and find confirmation of this change by the actions of others.

Wittreich and Radcliffe (1955) found that nondisabled men took a significantly greater amount of time to perceive simulated mutilation of the human figure than nonmutilated figures. They suggest that perception of a disabled person leads to an emotional response that is probably the reason for the lack of acceptance of disabled persons in society. Doob and Ecker (1970) found that housewives were more likely to comply with a request to fill out a questionnaire when the request was made by a stigmatized person (wearing a black eye patch) than by a nonstigmatized person. These researchers emphasize that these results hold for situations in which there is no further contact required between the stigmatized and nonstigmatized person. They do not know if such compliance would be obtained if compliance entailed further face-to-face interaction.

Kleck and his colleagues have conducted a series of studies regarding the effects of physical deviance on face-to-face interaction. Kleck, Ono, and Hastorf (1966) found that uncomfortableness, strangeness, and uncertainty in an interview situation lead to stereotyped and highly controlled behavior. The subjects interacting with an apparently physically disabled person demonstrated less variability in their behavior as a group, expressed opinions that were less representative of their actual beliefs, and terminated the interaction sooner than did subjects interacting with a nondisabled person. Kleck (1966) also found that subjects report less emotional confort when interacting with an apparently disabled person. In a further study, Kleck (1968) found that interactions with an apparently disabled person were associated with motoric inhibition, a more positive impression of the disabled person, and a distortion of opinion in the direction of making opinions more consistent with those assumed to be held by the disabled person. There was no difference in eye contact between the disabled-nondisabled interview and the nondisabled-nondisabled interview. These results were duplicated in another experiment which required longer interactions between apparently disabled and nondisabled persons, but the effects diminished slightly as interaction time increased (Kleck 1969).

Thus, Kleck interpreted these results as confirming Goffman's (1963) hypotheses about stigmatized persons. Interactions with stigmatized persons are avoided as much as possible and if interaction is necessary, the nondisabled person becomes somewhat emotionally aroused producing inhibited, constricted behavior. Nondisabled persons tend to become overly anxious to please the disabled person by complying with requests or shading their opinions to be consistent with what they think the disabled person believes.

An attempt to review the extensive literature on attitudes toward disabled persons will not be made in this document. However, for information on this topic, the review by English (1971) is recommended as a general introduction to this area. In addition, Wright (1960) has provided an excellent description of the psychosocial reactions to disabled persons and should be consulted for a more in-depth discussion of the issues presented in this chapter.

However, some of these issues can be summarized by comparing disabled persons to a minority group that is devalued in various ways. Wright (1960) believes that one characteristic of this minority group status is to be perceived as underprivileged and according to the stereotype of one who has suffered a great misfortune and whose life is consequently disturbed, distorted, and damaged. As a minority group, contact is avoided, thus preventing the nondisabled person from learning to behave more naturally around disabled persons.

Several studies have demonstrated that contact with and information about disabled persons can improve attitudes of the nondisabled toward the disabled. In fact, Anthony (1972) found that a combination of both contact and information is better than either of these alone. Clore and Jeffrey (1972) found that role playing (traveling around campus in a wheelchair) was an effective means of improving attitudes toward the disabled. Rapier and others (1972) found that integrating disabled children into classes with nondisabled children led the older children to develop more realistic attitudes about disabled children. Younger children were less realistic in their attitudes. Euse (1975) found that covert positive reinforcement was associated with improved attitudes and increased time spent looking at pictures of disabled persons.

Consequently, it appears that we all learn to perceive differences among people and to value those who are most physically attractive. We tend to avoid those who markedly deviate from our expectations and standards of appearance and, thus, do not learn how to behave in their presence. Initial contact with a disabled person apparently leads to anxiety, inhibited behavior, and attempts to please the person by complying with requests or giving opinions that are not necessarily our own but those we think will be consistent with those of the disabled person. However, contact with disabled people plus information about the disability appears to lead to more relaxed and natural social encounters.

FAMILY RELATIONSHIPS

There is no article or research project that deals with the reactions of parents to their teenagers or young adults who suffer spinal injury. What little has been written deals with issues of satisfaction within marriage for disabled groups in general and statistics on marriage and divorce among those with spinal injury.

Skipper, Fink, and Hallenbeck (1968) and Fink, Skipper, and Hallenbeck (1968) report the results of a study of marital relationships when the woman becomes disabled after marriage. They studied 36 disabled women and their husbands but did not report what types of disabilities were present in their sample. They found that there was little correlation between the husband's need for satisfaction and the degree of the wife's physical disability, and there was no relationship between degree of disability and total marital satisfaction. With high degrees of disability, however, the husband was less likely to feel companionship satisfaction. That is, while he got companionship at home, he did not have his wife's companionship on many outside physical activities that they used to share. Thus, the authors conclude that little can be predicted about a disabled woman's or her husband's marriage satisfaction on the knowledge of physical disability alone.

Klein, Dean, and Bogdonoff (1967) noted that the spouse of a chronically ill person will experience significant tension during the initial phases of the illness and that part of this tension is related to disruption of the usual roles each plays in marriage.

There have been references to role reversal which spinal injury may impose on married couples when the man acquires a spinal injury (Christopherson 1968; Dinsdale, Lesser, and Judd 1971), but we do not have any good data to assess this factor. Ludwig and Collette (1969) studied families of applicants for Social Security disability in Ohio and found that severely disabled men (many different disabilities) were less likely to respond positively to the item, "The man is always head of the household," than less severely disabled men. Fewer severely disabled men than less disabled computed the family income tax and made the decision on the purchase of a new car, but the low frequencies in each of these categories suggest that the base rates for this sample are for the wives to carry out these activities regardless of level of disability. Therefore, this study does not really assess the factor of role reversal and may be somewhat archaic in its definitions of sex roles in marriage. In any study of role reversal, we will have to determine the base rates of certain activities according to sex of the partner, and the age of the couple will probably be a significant factor in the outcome. Younger people and couples married more recently may display more equality and less rigidity in definition of the roles in a marriage than older couples. Socioeconomic status, ethnic group, and educational level may also be important variables in the outcome of such research. Thus, we will have to await future research before we can comment definitively on this factor of role reversal in marriages when one partner is disabled.

Many authors comment on the importance of the family in determining the outcome of our rehabilitation efforts. Harris and associates (1973) believe that the family determines the reaction of patients to their disability. Margolin (1971) reports unpublished data by Lowery indicating that the quality of the interpersonal relationships within the family are more important than the disability itself. Lowery proposes that if rehabilitation fails for no apparent reason, the family dynamics should be examined. If the family communicates an attitude of worth to the disabled person, his self-concept will be maintained, and he is more likely to participate in the rehabilitation process.

Litman (1962, 1964) studied 100 orthopedically disabled patients and found that those who were able to maintain a positive conception of self consistently responded to treatment, whereas those with negative self-conceptions tended to perform below expectations. Self-conception was defined as the person's evaluation of the attitudes of others toward himself as well as his sense of personal adequacy and worth. He also found that the degree of adjustment to the disabled role was a function of the degree of understanding the patient had as to what that role entailed. (This finding tends to challenge the strategy of rating adjustment to disability while the person is still hospitalized.) Litman found that family solidarity per se was not related to rehabilitation outcome, but amount of positive reinforcement received from the family was related to better performance in rehabilitation. Furthermore, patient performances seemed to be enhanced when therapy could be viewed in terms of reentry into an established family constellation. Previous social involvement also favored participation in rehabilitation activities as did a prior history of extensive physical activity.

Kerr and Thompson (1972) found that all the persons in their sample who were rated as having made an excellent mental adjustment to spinal injury had satisfactory lives prior to injury and most came from exceptionally warm and loving backgrounds. Kemp and Vash (1971) found that interpersonal support was positively correlated with degree of productivity in persons with quadriplegia, but this relationship did not hold for persons with paraplegia. And Cobb (1976), although not referring to physical disability per se, does emphasize the importance of social support as a moderator of life stresses in a large number of situations. He defines social support as information leading the person to believe that he is cared for or loved, and/or information leading a person to believe that he is esteemed and valued; and/or information leading the person to believe that he belongs to a network of communication and mutual obligation.

Persons with spinal injury have described the conflicts a disabled woman experiences and the difficulties that a family experiences when the woman is disabled. If there are children in the family, the mother with a disability often worries that she is asking too much of her children since she needs their assistance with many daily activities. Without children to help, it is difficult to manage all of the daily activities when the woman has quadriplegia, for example. The attendant will only do certain activities, and hired help will do only what they are told to do and usually no more. The family schedule revolves around the times that the attendant will be available to assist with the bowel program and this places significant constraints on a social life. Thus, spontaneity in social situations is very difficult. When the husband is employed or in school, there is great pressure on him to fill in at home with all of the extra chores that need to be done. Because she realizes how hard he is working at all of these tasks, the wife may feel that she cannot ask him for a favor since she has used up her ''allotment'' of requests, so to speak.

In addition, one key way of coping with a severe disability is to learn to minimize the problems and hassles, especially in regard to quadriplegia. This is not a denial, but rather a matter of orientation. There are so many difficulties that one needs to focus on the positive side of life and learn not to dwell on the inconveniences. However, this may lead to misunderstandings between a married couple as the disabled partner seems to be minimizing the difficulties involved in everyday life and the able-bodied partner is all too well aware of the difficulties. Therefore, open lines of communication are necessary for the survival of the marriage.

There are constant constraints on the freedom of the able-bodied partner which may add pressure in the relationship. The nondisabled partner may feel that he or she does not have as many options to be late from work or to stop for a beer with coworkers after work. There is a subtle sense of guilt and it is often self-imposed. The financial pressures of having to hire attendant and housekeeper services add to the difficulties of a marital relationship unless the able-bodied partner does not work and is prepared to do *this* work 24 hours a day for seven days a week, every year.

When the attendant suddenly quits, the able-bodied partner must perform the ADL and transfer activities that are necessary for survival. Many partners find that the bowel and bladder care are unpleasant and participation in such activities may possibly interfere with the quality of the relationship over time in some cases. The necessity of having attendant care available puts a constraint on any vacation planning unless the able-bodied partner is prepared to assume responsibility for these tasks while the couple is away (Consumer Conference 1977).

In a general sense, the process of mothering and fathering need not be influenced by severe disability. But, at young ages children need things done for them, and the mother with quadriplegia must watch while someone else puts the bandage on the skinned knee. The subtle competition that can arise between the housekeeper and the mother in regard to caring for the child will require great strength and social skill on the part of the disabled woman. In addition, if the couple choose to adopt a child, adoption agencies often reflect all of the prejudice and negative stereotypes of the disabled as found in the general population. Because of the disability, the agency assumes that it would be inappropriate to place a child in the family. Great efforts have to be made to convince the agency that this is not the case. However, Buck (1980) found that there was no difference in emotional adjustment or stability between a group of children raised by a disabled father and a group raised in a family without physical disability. There was no evidence that the disabled fathers excluded themselves from discipline and other child-rearing aspects of parenthood or that disabled fathers lose control over their children. In fact children of disabled fathers were found to hold significantly more positive attitudes toward their father than children of the nondisabled control group.

Comarr (1962, 1963) provides data on the marriage and divorce rate among veterans with spinal injury, but since these data may be somewhat out of date, the findings of El Ghatit and Hanson (1975 and 1976) who also studied United States veterans will be discussed. Apparently, their data overlap with that of Comarr's.

In a study of preinjury marriages, El Ghatit and Hanson found that 26.7 percent of the men who had been married at the time of injury were divorced at the time of the study. Of this group of divorced men, 76.4 percent reported that the injury had played a big role in the divorce. The authors note that the 26 percent divorce rate is lower than the base rate for the United States which is 33 percent and much lower than the base rate for divorce in California (the residence of most of the study sample) which is 50 percent. The divorce rate following onset of disability varied according to whether the person had ever been divorced prior to injury. Those in their first marriage at injury had a divorce rate of 27 percent, but those who had been married more than once had a divorce rate of 42 percent. Level of injury was not significantly related to incidence of divorce. The divorce rate was higher for couples who had preinjury and postinjury children in comparison to childless couples. This contradicts the impression that children have a stabilizing effect on marriages. Employment status was correlated with divorce rate. A lower divorce rate occurred in the men who had not been employed since injury or those who were employed at the time of the study. The highest divorce rate occurred in men who had been employed at some time postinjury but did not sustain the employment (37.7 percent). The lowest divorce rate occurred in those currently employed (17.6 percent).

Data on marriage and divorce after onset of spinal cord injury are supplied by El Ghatit and Hanson (1976). The overall divorce rate of those who had been single at injury was 24.6 percent. Of those divorced, only 41 percent thought that the spinal injury was a significant factor in the divorce in contrast to the 76 percent for divorces of preinjury marriages. This divorce rate is not significantly different from the divorce rate of preinjury marriages and also not significantly different from the overall United States divorce rate. Level of injury was significantly related to divorce rate of those who had been single at injury, persons with high thoracic lesions having the highest rate. However, considering all postinjury marriages, whether or not it was a remarriage, level of injury was not related to divorce rate. For those who were single at injury, the presence of postinjury children (whether natural or adopted) was associated with a significantly lower divorce rate (7.4 percent) in comparison to those who had no children living with them (25 percent). The presence of children was not related to divorce rate in persons who remarried after injury.

Interestingly, those who remained single even after injury were less likely to have improved their educational status than those who were married. However, postinjury education was not related to divorce rate. In addition, males who remained single were less likely to obtain employment than those who were married. But of those who did obtain postinjury employment, those who were single were more likely to sustain the employment. No relationship between current employment and divorce rate was found for postinjury marriages.

Deyoe (1972a) reports data on marriage among United States veterans in the northeastern part of the U.S. and claims that there was a greater stability for marriages contracted following injury. Also, he states that there was no difference between the veterans with service-connected versus non-service-connected disabilities in divorce rate, but he does not provide data on this factor.

Information on the marriages of a civilian, nonveteran population, has been collected by Crewe, Athelstan, and Krumberger (1978). Of the 128 persons with spinal injury who had been interviewed in depth, 35 had been married at the time of their injury and 35 married since the injury. Eleven of the preinjury marriages ended in divorce and 4 of the postinjury marriages failed. However, there was a great difference in the longevity of the marriages and the average age of the two groups, the preinjury group being older and married longer. Nevertheless, the median length of marriage in the postinjury group was five years.

Comparisons of the marriages that occurred prior to injury and after injury revealed that the disabled person was viewed as a contributing member of the family in both groups and not as a burden. However, psychologists' assessments of the marriages based on the in-depth interviews indicated that the postinjury marriages seemed happier and the spouses seemed more satisfied in comparison to the preinjury group. In marriages contracted preinjury, the disabled partner was more likely to have unnecessary help with daily activities and one-third of the preinjury group claimed to be satisfied with no sexual activity at all, whereas only one of the postinjury marital units made such a response. Those in the postinjury marital group were more likely to be employed than those married prior to injury. Interestingly, those married preinjury who had successful marriages were more likely to be farmers and live in a rural or small town area. Those who married after injury tended to live in a city.

Because of the nature of their study, Crewe and her associates collected little information about the marriages that ended but report that all persons involved in failed marriages were urban residents; none were farmers before injury. Five of the 6 women who were married at time of injury were later divorced in comparison to 6 out of 29 men who became divorced. The small number of women in the study does not permit any conclusion to be drawn, but the authors suggest that a marriage may be more fragile when the woman becomes the disabled partner.

Although we need more data on this issue, special attention should be given to women with spinal injury. We have some tentative evidence that their marriages may not be as likely to succeed following disability, and there is the clinical impression that single, disabled women may be less likely to get married following injury. We need research to determine the validity of this impression and we need to give disabled women the opportunity for intensive social skills training to help them counteract the prejudice that some men have about dating a woman with a disability.

Future research on this issue should be possible using data collected by the National Spinal Cord Injury Data Research Center in Phoenix, Arizona. Researchers should consider the El Ghatit and Hanson studies as a model of how the data should be analyzed. Detailed statistical analyses are necessary in order to assess the multitude of variables that are associated with divorce. It is recommended that the style of these authors be followed, i.e., the data be considered separately for those who have been married preinjury and those who contract their first marriage following injury. The financial security of the couple should be assessed because Kerr and Thompson (1972) found that this was an important factor in the adjustment to spinal injury.

Clinical impression suggests that those marriages that are unstable prior to injury will be further stressed by the injury. Does this group have the highest divorce rate? Are marriages contracted after injury more stable? El Ghatit and Hanson say no and Deyoe says yes. What are the stresses on a marriage when spinal injury hits one partner? We have no data. Is role reversal a problem and how do we define it? Are females who are single at onset of spinal injury less likely to contract a marriage than males because of the double standard regarding physical attractiveness? What is the role of culture and ethnic group on marriages among those with spinal injury? Do men of some ethnic groups reject their wives who sustain a spinal injury because they fear that their masculine image is hurt? Are women of some ethnic groups less likely to marry a man with spinal injury? There are many questions to which we have no answer. In addition, we must ask if there are strategies that would be successful in assisting the person with spinal injury to cope with the complicated social world outside of the rehabilitation center.

DEMOGRAPHIC VARIABLES

There is some evidence to support clinical intuition that certain demographic variables, along with severity of disability, may influence the process of adjustment to spinal cord injury in certain individuals. Thus, we will examine the literature to determine what we know and do not know about the influence of age at onset, severity of disability, duration of disability, socioeconomic status, sex, ethnic background, urban-rural residence, and financial security.

Age

Data from the National Spinal Cord Injury Data Research Center in Phoenix, Arizona (Young 1977; National Spinal Cord Injury Model Systems Conference 1978), confirms our suspicion that spinal cord injury affects the young. The data indicates that injuries resulting in paraplegia are most likely to occur to persons age 30 or under. Sixty-seven percent of those with paraplegia were injured at age 30 or less, the most frequent age group being ages 15–20 which has 27 percent of the cases. The data is even more striking for persons with quadriplegia, 62 percent of the injuries occurring in persons under age 25, with the most frequent age group being ages 15–20 (34 percent). Spinal injury occurs after age 45 in only 9.3 percent of the total cases according to this national sample.

Wilcox and Stauffer (1972) followed 423 persons from Rancho Los Amigos Hospital and looked at what happened by age category. Of those who were over age 40 at injury, 25 percent were dead at follow-up in contrast to 9 percent death rate in those injured between ages 14 to 19 years. They note, however, that the group aged 20 to 40 at injury seemed to have the greatest amount of troubles. In this age group occurred the most suicides, the highest incidence of unlawful behavior prior to injury, and the highest percentage of persons living in nursing homes. The employment rate was 3 percent higher than for the younger group, but the college enrollment rate was 20 percent lower than the younger group. Wilcox and Stauffer state:

> This middle group reflects some habits of both extremes. Some are still being propelled forward by their individual life-styles; some seem to have had their early aspirations blunted by exposure to the world after leaving home and before they became fully established as independent adults. They of the three groups appear to be the most vulnerable to tragedy and the least predictable, and defied categorization in this study. (Wilcox and Stauffer 1972, p. 121)

Kerr and Thompson (1972) followed 181 persons with spinal injury and rated them on their mental adjustment to the spinal cord injury (methodology of rating is unspecified). They found that 83 percent of those aged 10–20 made a good or excellent adjustment, 61 percent of those aged 20–45, and 41 percent of those over 45. Fifty-one percent of those over 45 who were rated as not having adjusted were dead at time of follow-up. Regarding the 20–45 age group, the authors conclude that differences in personality and home circumstances seemed to play very important roles in determining outcomes. Thus Kerr and Thompson conclude that age is a very important factor, the young adjusting better than the old.

Hallin (1968) noted that whereas level of lesion had a great effect on independence, age did also. This was especially apparent in the incomplete quadriplegic category. Older persons with incomplete quadriplegia were less likely to be independent in function than their younger counterparts.

Dinsdale, Lesser, and Judd (1971) divide their patients into three categories according to constellation of problems presented. They believe that the young male has the most difficult adjustment problems as defined by the number of problems listed using the Problem Oriented Medical Record approach. However, they do not have follow-up data to determine whether there is a correlation between number of potential problems identified during inpatient rehabilitation and number of actual problems following discharge. Judging by the data of Wilcox and Stauffer and Kerr and Thompson, this group might do very well.

Ludwig and Adams (1968) noted that the very young and very old were more likely to complete rehabilitation services than the intermediate age group. They interpret this in terms of ease in assuming the client role by those who already are in dependent or subordinate social roles outside of the hospital.

Kemp and Vash (1971) found an interaction between age and number of reported goals. Among those reporting a high number of goals, the younger individuals were more productive and the older persons were somewhat less productive.

Consequently, there seems to be some consensus that the very young may have a less difficult time adapting to the changed life circumstances that disability requires. Onset before age 20 seems to be associated with somewhat better adjustment on the whole than later onset although there are tremendous individual differences. Using the national data on spinal injury (presented in figure 1.2), 29.54 percent of the injuries occur before age 20, 36.96 percent between ages 20 and 29, and 33.5 percent at age 30 and over. It is not that age per se is the factor, but more likely it is the social psychological stage of adulthood that accounts for the differences.

The research by Levinson, Darrow, Klein, Levinson, and McKee (1978) and Sheehy's book *Passages* (1974 and 1976) may provide some interesting clues as to the types of adjustments that a nondisabled person is making at various points in adult life, which then become additional pressures at the time of disability. In essence, it appears that the ages 20 through 35 are very formative years as the person establishes an identity and creates a role for himself that provides the opportunity for self-acceptance and stability later in life. Within this context, those injured before age 20, may not have begun or gotten very far into this process and, therefore, they can establish an identity in which the disability becomes an integral part of who they are. Within the twenties and thirties, however, there may be more readjustment required of the newly disabled person and for this group "inner strength" and all that this implies is a more critical variable. Disability after age 40 might produce two groups: those who "give up" and those who still have some important items on their agenda, so to speak. In these latter two age groups, one might speculate that those with an internal locus of control would be more successful than externals. This is a question for research; however, the evidence suggests that we should give more than passing attention to age of onset as a factor in adjustment to spinal injury.

Severity of Disability

Quadriplegia imposes greater limitations on a person than paraplegia, and the question then arises as to whether persons with quadriplegia, on the average, are less well adjusted than paraplegics. Therefore, we will examine any study that provides information related to severity of disability.

Ludwig and Adams (1968) found that severity of disability was a factor associated with the completion of rehabilitation services and discuss the data in terms of the ability to assume the client role which entails some degree of dependence and subordination. However, in the case of severe disability, it may be that the person believes that he has fewer options and, therefore, must complete the services in order to attain as much skill as possible. Unquestionably, a person with less severe disability can quit a rehabilitation program and still do well if he chooses.

Seymour (1955) studied the social and personal adjustment of persons with paraplegia and quadriplegia. Social adjustment was rated by ward staff on an instrument designed for the study. No validity data was presented. Personal adjustment was judged by blind analyses of Rorschach protocols. She found that persons with quadriplegia were rated as more socially adjusted than those with paraplegia. There was no difference in personal adjustment between these two groups. She comments, however, that the adjectives applied to those judged to be socially adjusted were "compliant," "cooperative," "gives little trouble," "is quiet," "is nice," which may not be "a desirable situation from the standpoint of good psychological health" (Seymour 1955, p. 693). This study was conducted in the early 1950s on a Veterans Administration hospital population. No information on duration of the disability is given and one wonders if the persons with quadriplegia were living in the hospital rather than receiving initial rehabilitation services. Therefore, these data must be treated with caution. However, we can say that the persons with quadriplegia had, indeed, identified what behavior was necessary in order to get along with the staff on whom their survival depended.

Cull and Smith (1973) found that incidence of decubitus ulcers was unrelated to any of the variables they studied except sex. Males were more likely to experience skin breakdowns than women. Severity of disability was not a factor. However, Anderson and Andberg (1977), in a truly excellent study, found that as a group, persons with quadriplegia had a lower incidence of pressure sores than the group with paraplegia.

Hohmann (1966) found a tendency for the experience of emotional feelings to be reduced with increasing severity of disability. Jasnos and Hakmiller (1975) report that persons with cervical lesions were less responsive to sexual stimuli than persons with lower lesions. However, this study can be criticized on methodological grounds and the results must be considered tentative. At this time there is no evidence that a reduction in experienced emotional feelings is an advantage or disadvantage in adjusting to spinal injury. Therefore, this becomes a question for research.

Kemp and Vash (1971) found a significant interaction between level of injury and interpersonal support as factors in productivity. With high interpersonal support, there was no difference between persons with paraplegia and quadriplegia. But with less support, persons with quadriplegia were significantly less productive.

Meyerson (1968) reports that internal versus external locus of control is not related to level of injury. Dinardo (1971) notes that those with severe disabilities are somewhat more depressed than those with less severe disabilities regardless of their locus of control or position on the repressor-sensitizer dimension. Among those with less severe disabilities, internal repressors are less depressed than external sensitizers. Swenson (1976) found that locus of control and satisfaction with life were unrelated to level of disability.

And finally there is a study by Golightly and Reinehr (1972) that questions whether the psychological environment and the reality of the disability might be very different for persons with quadriplegia versus paraplegia. They wondered if those with quadriplegia become psychologically different from those with less severe disabilities and the nondisabled. Thus, they administered the Holtzman Inkblot Technique to 16 persons with quadriplegia who were residents of a domiciliary workshop. These persons had been receiving custodial care before entry into the workshop program. They describe the results in these terms:

> The subjects in the present sample are least like college students and most like 5-year olds in their pattern of responses to the inkblots. They are also rather more similar to the ''pathological'' groups (Schizophrenics, Mentally Retarded, Depressed patients) than to the ''normal'' groups. (Golightly and Reinehr 1972, p. 48)

The question that these researchers planned to study is an interesting one and it is too bad that they did not test the question. An alternative and highly probable interpretation of their data is that they reflect the effects of social and psychological stagnation which extended institutionalization can produce no matter what the disability might be. The authors give no information on duration of disability, length of institutionalization, age, or the reasons that these persons were not out in the community. They observe that it is difficult, if not impossible, to obtain an adequate control group for their sample which seems to be an implicit recognition on their part of the unrepresentativeness of their group to the population with quadriplegia. Otherwise, a sample of persons with paraplegia would be nice as a minimum, in addition to a sample of persons without spinal injury who have been institutionalized for a similar (but unspecified) period of time. Another control group would be a sample of able-bodied subjects who have been participants in a sensory deprivation experiment. Although the authors admit that this is a preliminary investigation and that "only limited inferences can be drawn from such crude data" (Golightly and Reinehr 1972, p. 48), we do not believe that such disclaimers reduce the obligation that researchers have to submit for publication only those works having some degree of methodological soundness as a basis for interpretation of the results. Golightly-Eberly (1978) fully concurs with these observations and regrets that the study was published.

Thus, in terms of severity of disability, there is no evidence that higher levels of injury and greater functional limitation lead to a poorer adjustment to spinal cord injury. One wonders if the physical and psychological reality of quadriplegia versus paraplegia leads to differences in *how* one adapts (although level of adjustment could be similar depending upon the person and the environment), and this is a question to be tested in the future. Nagler (1950) discusses quadriplegia as a separate reaction type, but we have no evidence that this is, in fact, the case. One wonders if persons with quadriplegia need to develop a greater skill at coping with interpersonal relationships than persons with paraplegia because the former group's very survival often depends upon their ability to get along with those around them. However, future research into spinal cord injury should specify the level of injury or severity of disability so that we can test some of these questions.

Duration of Disability

We talk about the *process* of adjustment to disability and believe that it occurs over a period of many years. Carter (1977) and Kerr and Thompson (1972) believe that at least two years are needed before the person achieves some sense of stability in his life. However, amazingly enough, there is no data to document this course of adjustment to spinal cord injury. Very little of our data is longitudinal in nature, and many studies in the literature do not even specify the duration of disability of persons in their samples. When researchers do specify duration, the average duration is given and, from the range, one knows that the standard deviation must be high. Can we assume that the reactions of a person injured for six months are similar to the reactions of someone injured for five years?

Longitudinal research is needed to study this issue. Willems (1976a, 1976b) and his associates have been following a series of persons with spinal injury for a number of years, but data are not yet available on the long-term adjustment of these people. This issue requires study by other researchers, but, in the meanwhile, all studies should specify duration of disability and reduce the size of the standard deviation of this parameter.

Sex

Data from the National Spinal Cord Injury Data Research Center (Young 1977) indicates that approximately 20 percent of the spinal injuries occur in women, but there is a slight difference in incidence of paraplegia and quadriplegia. In a national sample of 1,687 cases injured between 1973 and 1976, we have the following information:

	Paraplegia	Quadriplegia	Total
Male	649 (79.3%)	727 (83.7%)	1,376 (81.6%)
Female	169 (20.7%)	142 (16.3%)	311 (18.4%)
Total	818 (100.0%)	869 (100.0%)	1,687 (100.0%)

It appears that 54 percent of the women who are injured incur paraplegia and 46 percent sustain a quadriplegia, whereas, in men, 47 percent become paraplegic and 53 percent become quadriplegic.

Most of the studies do not refer to the sex of the persons with spinal cord injury and the number of women in any sample would admittedly be small. However, Kutner and Kutner (1979) found that in a group of southern men and women, men missed their independence and their job most and women reported losses in interpersonal relationships following disability. It would be interesting to cross-validate these findings on a larger sample and one that included northern, urban residents. Other than this study, there is little data as to whether women react differently to spinal injury than men, and until this issue is studied, it is not appropriate to group all persons with spinal injury together into one unisex category. Since women, according to our records, do account for 18 percent of the total sample, it seems appropriate to study this issue. However, since 82 percent of the spinal injuries occur in men and most of the data reported is based on samples of males, the masculine pronouns have been used in this document in a generic sense for the purpose of convenience and simplicity. This usage of language should not be interpreted to suggest that we believe that women are less worthy of consideration on any of the issues discussed in this document.

Socioeconomic Status and Culture

Socioeconomic status (SES) can influence the reaction to spinal cord injury in several ways: it has played a role in shaping the person's personality style up to the point of injury, and it correlates highly with the environmental resources that the person has available to him as he faces the world as a person with a disability.

Lefcourt (1976) reports that SES correlates with locus of control. Persons from less affluent or deprived backgrounds are more likely to perceive that the world's resources are outside of their control. The person sees himself as a victim of fate, luck, or chance, and tends to have an external locus of control. This personality factor may be a very important one in the ultimate adjustment to spinal cord injury. Amount of education and attitude toward education may vary according to SES and this may be a very influential factor on outcome after spinal cord injury. Consequently, all of the parameters of SES should be investigated and related to adjustment to spinal cord injury.

Meyerson (1968) found that race was one of the few factors that correlated with his measure of locus of control. Blacks were more external than whites. Kalb (1971) reported that social class and incidence of depression predicted postdischarge outcomes. Persons of a lower SES who were depressed did poorly after discharge. Ludwig and Adams (1968) found that nonwhites, the unemployed, and those referred by public agencies were persons most likely to complete rehabilitation services. They interpret these data in terms of ability to assume a dependent and subordinate role. Kerr and Thompson (1972) found that examples of good adjustment to spinal injury were found in all social classes in their sample. But they report that persons in the best-adjusted category had more education than those in the less-adjusted categories. Furthermore, they state that financial hardship was certainly a deterrent to good adjustment. In 30 cases rated as excellent in adjustment, there was only one in which financial hardship might have been a problem.

Culture and ethnic background play a similar role to SES; they influence the person prior to injury and continue to do so afterward. Spinal injured males from cultures in which masculinity is equated with physical prowess, success with females, and fathering of many children may have a more difficult time in adjusting to spinal injury. True or false?

There are many issues affecting a person's life that may correlate with adjustment to spinal injury. But there is little data to document these influences. Consequently, future research should specify the nature of the subject population more precisely so that we can begin to assess the role of socioeconomic status and culture as factors in the adjustment to spinal cord injury.

Urban-Rural Residence

We can speculate as to the advantages and disadvantages of urban versus rural residence, but there is little data available to determine if this is a factor in outcome after spinal cord injury other than that offered by Crewe, Athelstan, and Krumberger (1978) regarding success of preinjury marriages. Urban areas may have more resources for medical attention and for education and social outlets (if they are physically accessible), but cities may be lonely places with greater social isolation than small communities. Rural areas may provide more interpersonal support and the historical ties to the region may cover several generations in contrast to urban residents. Whether these environmental factors are influential in the ultimate adjustment to spinal injury, we do not know. Thus, this becomes another area for research.

THE TASK OF SOCIALIZATION

Kahn (1969) notes that the current system of medical care does not improve the self-esteem of anyone with spinal injury.

> Current medical care is structured to gain control of the patient through depersonalization and infantilization, which reinforce the regression in social functioning that occurs in any illness experience, let alone one of catastrophic dimensions. The patient's already shaken self image is further weakened when he is tagged for identification and divested of his clothes and other personal belongings, and when he realizes that others are planning his daily schedule. His control and right to privacy seem to vanish as he becomes open territory for any member of the medical team who wants to ask him questions or to examine him. His self image is further damaged by hospital personnel who call him by his first name and coax him as though he were a child. (Kahn 1969, pp. 757-58)

Using the analogy of physical rehabilitation, Kahn goes on to point out the necessity of preventing social problems, just as we focus on preventing pressure sores, contractures, and kidney and bladder stones. The patient must be involved in all planning and decision making, and the family should be included in all phases of the treatment.

Weissman and Kutner (1967) elaborate on these ideas and discuss, in detail, the role disorders that may develop with extended hospitalization. The disabled person can become overly preoccupied with himself because of the monotony and constricting nature of hospital environments. He is unable to influence his environment because most hospitals permit little individuality in decision making. Thus, the hospital may unintentionally undermine social competence since there is little opportunity to practice social skills. Basically, the person with a disability is in a subordinate position throughout the hospitalization and, thus, would feel very unskilled at coping with the devaluation he will experience after discharge. The patient-patient relationships are tenuous and transitory, and the hospital routine does interfere with the close personal contact between intimates. During the hospitalization, he is on a leave of absence, so to speak, from his job, school, and social life. Consequently, all of these factors, these realities of hospitalization, impinge on a person at a time when he himself questions his self-image.

The hospitalization process does have positive features, however. Spinal cord injury centers provide the newly injured person with models and peers so that he need not feel so tremendously isolated from others. In addition, the basic survival skills will be learned in a supportive and encouraging atmosphere. Thus, the question becomes, can we modify our present procedures to enhance later social functioning or should we introduce social skills training as part of the rehabilitation process. Perhaps we should try both.

Cogswell (1967, 1968) points out that in contrast to the sheltered social environment of hospital and home, the community is a setting where the real and perceived stigma of disability reach their height of salience. Salience of stigma varies with the type of social other and type of social setting, with the person's definition and projection of self as worthy or demeaned, and with his skill in managing others' definitions of him. Thus, persons with spinal injury may reduce the stigmatizing effects of disability by limiting social encounters to others and social settings where they feel the stigma is less salient, by projecting a definition of self as worthy, which tends to counter negative definitions by others, and by becoming skilled in eliciting positive definitions of self from others.

Cogswell hypothesizes that following discharge, persons with spinal injury tend to phase out relationships with pretrauma friends, develop new friendships with lower status others, and then finally acquire new friends of similar pretrauma status. She believes that situations in which both persons have social handicaps allow the person with the disability to have the opportunity to experiment with new behavior in less threatening situations. The person with a new spinal injury will select social settings depending on the physical accessibility, the flexibility for leaving the scene, and the salience of the stigma. She further categorizes physical accessibility (in order of ease) as those settings where the person can go and remain in his car; those allowing easy wheelchair maneuvering; those that can be easily entered by wheelchair but require a transfer out of the wheelchair to a different seat; those in which physical assistance is required in order to enter the setting.

This outline of the socialization process, presented by Cogswell (1967, 1968), seems to be based on her observations of and interviews with a series of persons with spinal injury. She does not present data, and, therefore, the above must be considered to be hypotheses about the process of socialization that might be the subject of research. She defines socialization as a continuous process of learning to abandon old roles and self-conceptions and to acquire new ones, and she chastises sociologists for attempting to study socialization as a static phenomenon rather than a dynamic process. The same criticism can be applied to psychologists and other researchers; therefore, longitudinal research seems to be the most appropriate technique to enhance our knowledge of the changes that occur following spinal injury.

However, an example of good cross-sectional research was performed by Mesch (1976) who studied the content of verbal interactions between college students with spinal injury and with no disability. She found that dyads consisting of two nondisabled partners exhibited the least amount of self-disclosure at all levels of topic intimacy, while dyads consisting of two disabled partners exhibited the greatest amount of self-disclosure on low and medium intimacy topics. The mixed dyads, consisting of one disabled and one nondisabled partner, exhibited the greatest amount of self-disclosure on the high intimacy topic. She states that in the mixed dyads, the subjects appeared interested in each other but proceeded cautiously using the experimental task as a vehicle for getting to know each other. The quality of the interaction appeared to be partially dependent on the degree to which the disabled subject could establish rapport with his nondisabled partner. In dyads in which a positive interaction occurred, the disabled partner demonstrated initiative in volunteering information, openness about himself and his experience, and responsiveness to his partner's disclosures.

Davis (1961) provides an excellent sociological analysis of the interaction process between a disabled and nondisabled person based on interviews with 11 socially skilled, visibly handicapped persons. These informants substantiate the observations by Mesch that the success of the interaction is usually a function of the skill with which the disabled person puts the nondisabled person at ease. The person with a disability must learn techniques to overcome the initial strain in the interaction and must find ways of establishing rapport so that the nondisabled person can learn to forget the presence of the disability.

Consequently, the person with spinal injury faces a formidable task. Not only must he learn to mobilize himself and function despite the motor and sensory loss, but he must learn to put people at ease. Unfortunately, rehabilitation centers have emphasized those tasks relating to physical functioning and have essentially ignored those tasks relating to social functioning.

Romano (1976) has called for increased social skills training for the newly handicapped as a means of ensuring success of our rehabilitation efforts. She describes social competence as those adaptive verbal and action skills that permit people to have some control over their interactions with others. This training would recognize an individual's strengths and use behavioral rehearsal and assignment in which a person considers a given situation, identifies the alternative types of responses, and practices a chosen response in a situation which provides him with feedback. Although data are not presented, Romano states that patients who have participated in social skills training during rehabilitation hospitalization report that they enter social situations more readily and with less anxiety after discharge.

It is recommended that social skills training become an integral part of all rehabilitation programs and that research be conducted to assess its value. In this chapter, the various factors that complicate the social life of the individual following spinal injury or any disability have been described, but there has been little definitive research in this area. We must specify the behaviors that a person with spinal injury needs in order to cope with nondisabled persons and teach these skills as part of rehabilitation. Whether these skills should be included as part of the inpatient rehabilitation program or should be considered to be a second phase in the rehabilitation process should be studied. At this time, there are some attempts to include transitional living experiences during the inpatient rehabilitation phase.

Manley and Armstrong (1976) describe the use of a transitional living facility at one of the regional spinal injury centers. During the last two weeks of rehabilitation, the patients are requested to reside in an apartment complex with their families in order to test the skills and techniques learned in the rehabilitation program. The patients are still under the supervision of the hospital staff so that problems can be identified and corrected and self-confidence can grow before actual discharge. They report that those discharged after the transitional living experience have fewer medical complications and social crises than patients discharged without this experience.

In the last several years, there have developed centers for independent living run by the disabled for the disabled. Peer counseling regarding daily life experiences has been included and is another attempt to fill the gap between the physical skills learned in the traditional rehabilitation center and the skills needed to cope with the world. Some of these programs have residential facilities and others do not. These programs will be discussed in more detail in chapter 8.

RECREATION

The onset of spinal injury may interfere with a certain number of recreational activities that a person had enjoyed prior to injury, especially if these activities involved physical performance. Since recreation is part of everyone's life in some form and is viewed as essential for reducing tension and offsetting the hard work of daily life, it is especially important in the life of a person with a disability. Since 80 percent of spinal injuries occur to males and a large proportion of them are young, recreation can provide some rewards and opportunities for physical activity and even competition which was a part of their life prior to injury.

Guttmann (1976) has recognized the importance of recreation, and athletic competition, in the lives of persons with spinal injury. He believes that sports can improve physiological functioning and can be a means of maintaining cardiopulmonary conditioning and general health. Strength, endurance, and coordination may improve as the result of participation in athletic activities. Furthermore, he believes that, in addition to the physical benefits, athletics have psychological and social benefits as well. Participation in sports activities can be one means of developing self-confidence and can become one avenue through which the person can reenter community life.

Annually, competitions are held at Stoke Mandeville Hospital in England and during Olympic years these competitions are held, if possible, in the same country as the Olympic Games. National and regional competitions are held around the United States and many have endorsed recreation as an important part of a rehabilitation program (Crase 1972; Lynch 1972; Sheredos 1973; Jochheim and Strohkindl 1973; Robinson 1973). The advantages of horseback riding for persons with disabilities has been mentioned, and swimming is favored by others (Tomita and Matsubayashi 1964; Geis 1975). Guttmann and Mehra (1973) are particularly impressed with the value of archery since it may be one of the only sports in which the disabled person can compete on equal terms with able-bodied persons.

Martial arts may be another area that might be rewarding to persons with disabilities. Able-bodied persons report an increase in self-confidence as a result of such training. Thus, this should be included as an option for persons with disabilities.

Since everyone needs a reason for getting out of bed in the morning, recreational activities should be a legitimate part of a rehabilitation program. The purpose of these activities should not only be entertainment, but rather they should be considered to be therapeutic activities. They should focus on teaching the person with the disability skills that he might find rewarding later in life.

It would be interesting to compare two groups of persons: those with no recreational training and those given significant training and opportunity to practice a sport of their choice. Does the latter group participate in a wider variety of activities following discharge than the group without such training? This should be tested.

AGING

At this time within the history of the treatment of spinal injury, we are approaching an issue that has never before been a concern. That population of persons who sustained their spinal cord injuries during World War II are approximately age 50 and are facing changes in their lives that are similar to those in the able-bodied population of a similar age. The concerns about role in life, retirement, and declining physical capacity will be similar to those of the able-bodied person, but we do not know if there will be differences that spinal injury introduces to the situation.

Hohmann (1978b) points out that the person with spinal injury may begin to worry about his longevity and wonder if he will have time to do the things in life he would like. The concern about independence and physical function may lead to worries about nursing home placement if the spouse is not capable of helping the disabled person any longer. In turn, will the disabled person be able to assist the able-bodied spouse if illness or disability strikes? Furthermore, concerns about the financial security of the spouse and children arise, especially since disability pensions decline or cease upon death of the disabled partner. It would seem, then, that approaching seniority reintroduces concern about issues that might have been resolved somewhat up to that point but which are always core issues in the life of the disabled person: physical function, independence, relationship to family members, and financial security.

These concerns should be the focus of research. Within the Veterans Administration there should be ample opportunity to gather data on these issues. Furthermore, the National Spinal Cord Injury Data Research Center should monitor these issues, particularly those regarding declining physical function with age.

SUMMARY

The onset of spinal injury changes a person's social stimulus value, and this change will be reflected in almost all areas of life. The world is designed for and populated by able-bodied people who become constricted and uncomfortable in the presence of a person with a disability. The success of the disabled person's social interactions largely depends on his ability to assert himself, to initiate contact, and to put the other person at ease. This requires a large repertoire of social skills which he usually must learn by himself. Some never learn to be socially skillful, and their productivity may be limited as a result. We need to introduce social skills training as a part of the rehabilitation program and we need to develop research programs documenting the outcomes of these efforts.

Research shows that several demographic variables may influence response to spinal injury. Youth favors a good adjustment, but there are significant individual differences. Duration of disability and severity of disability are factors that need to be investigated, yet we have no evidence to date that these are factors in adjustment to spinal injury. Sex may be a factor, but females account for only 18 percent of the spinal injury population and may not be present in that proportion in any one sample. However, until this is studied, we should not assume a homogeneity of reaction to spinal injury. Socioeconomic status has been implicated in several studies as being a factor that influences outcome, but this, too, needs to be investigated further.

We have not discussed the issue of changing the attitudes of society toward the disabled person through programs of education or advertising. Rather, we believe that focusing our efforts on enhancing the social skills of the individual with a disability may be the more productive route toward accomplishing such changes. If able-bodied people have some successful interactions with disabled people, these successful experiences may lead to greater changes in attitudes than an educational program with no contact.

If persons with disabilities become more skillful in social interactions, their visibility will be increased and, perhaps, their productivity will also be increased. Thus, a key research priority for the future must be the development of strategies to teach social skills to persons with spinal injury and to promote programs of research to assess the outcomes.

5
Variables Associated with Productivity Following Spinal Cord Injury

Neff (1971) believes that one of the more curious and significant aspects of the rehabilitation movement in the United States has been the closeness of its ties to issues relating to work and employment. The goals of rehabilitation have gone beyond those of medical restoration to those of assisting the disabled person to adapt as much as possible to the demands of social living. Furthermore, there has always been in our society a heavy emphasis on gainful employment as a condition for full citizenship.

> The interaction of these two components, further reinforced by the explicit mission of a federal agency chiefly responsible for the funding of rehabilitation programs, has brought about a situation where *rehabilitation* and *vocational rehabilitation* are virtually synonymous terms (Neff 1971, p. 113)

As a result, successful rehabilitation has been defined, by departments of rehabilitation, as a full-time employment for at least 60 days. Anything less than this has been considered to reflect failure. However, if we use this as our definition of success in working with persons who have a spinal injury, we will have to come to the conclusion that we have not been very successful as the statistics cited below will demonstrate.

Consequently, it is a thesis of this chapter that *a successful life consists of many types of behaviors, and employment is only one of these*. As a result, it is more appropriate and realistic to talk about productivity in all of its dimensions, rather than to focus exclusively on employment. Furthermore, many persons with spinal injury would like to express themselves through work but find that there are too many obstacles preventing them from doing so.

DEFINITION OF PRODUCTIVITY

In a previous report, Trieschmann (1971, 1974) proposed that there were three categories of functioning associated with a successful life, whether or not one is disabled. The first category is the *prevention of medical complications and the utilization of ADL mobility skills*. Either the person takes care of himself or he operates on his environment in such a manner that assures that he will be given proper care. A second category entails the *maintenance of a stable living environment*. Required here are all of the social skills that we use in order to cope with society, family, friends, and one's attendant. A third category is *productivity* which may entail vocational endeavors, education, volunteer activities, and avocational pursuits. Swenson (1976) in a follow-up study that utilized these categories as his outcome variables found that locus of control correlated with performance in each of these categories. However, he substituted satisfaction with life for category two, maintenance of a stable living environment. Each of the above categories is applicable to each person to some degree. Success would be defined as functioning at the maximum level at which one is capable. Success, then, has a flexible definition depending on the unique combination of circumstances surrounding each case. In this way, we avoid the pitfall of forming a rigid and absolute definition of success which is applied to each person with spinal injury regardless of his circumstances. Furthermore, with this conceptualization of success, our rehabilitation efforts can be focused on the process of living rather than on one parameter of a person's life.

Many professionals have expressed concern about the inadequacy of criteria of psychological and social outcomes, and there is agreement that no single measure can describe the complex nature of adjustment to spinal cord injury. This concern is shared by Kemp and Vash (1971) who studied the productivity of persons with spinal cord injury. They define productivity as activities of a constructive nature including avocational pursuits, group participation, and family responsibilities, in addition to employment. Deyoe (1972b), in a follow-up study of veterans, notes that although a small proportion of his sample is involved in gainful employment, a large proportion of the sample is involved in a great number of different activities. Thus he describes his group as gainfully productive, rather than gainfully employed. Finally, Kerr and Thompson (1972) note that a satisfactory return to work of some kind is more likely to be the result of good adjustment than a factor in achieving it. Consequently, there is great concern about the appropriateness of using employment as the single measure of rehabilitation success, and the data on employment following spinal cord injury will demonstrate the validity of these concerns.

DATA ON EMPLOYMENT

It is difficult to find a report that describes employment figures for persons with spinal injury that does not contain some bias. Some reports include individuals with other than traumatic spinal cord injury, and some are heavily influenced by self-selection of the subjects which is a problem in questionnaire studies. Thus, for a picture of the employment situation of a fairly unbiased sample of persons with spinal injury, we will have to await data from the National Spinal Cord Data Research Center in Phoenix, Arizona.

Brown and Chanin (1974) and Chanin and Brown (1975) report data on clients with spinal injury for fiscal year 1972–73 who were closed from plan by the California State Department of Rehabilitation. Out of a total of 117 cases, 48 percent were rehabilitated (employed for 60 days or more), and 52 percent were not rehabilitated. Of those rehabilitated, 75 percent were persons with paraplegia and 25 percent with quadriplegia. Of those not rehabilitated, 59 percent had a diagnosis of paraplegia and 41 percent quadriplegia. Within the category of paraplegia, 54 percent were rehabilitated and 46 percent were not. Within the category of quadriplegia, 36 percent were rehabilitated and 64 percent were not. There was no difference in age between the successful and unsuccessful cases, but educational levels both at referral and closure were different. More of the rehabilitated clients entered the rehabilitation process with some education beyond high school as compared to nonrehabilitated clients. At closure, 41 percent of the rehabilitated clients had earned at least a bachelor's degree in college whereas only 7 percent of the nonrehabilitated clients had done so. Interestingly, they found that a major reason for non-rehabilitation was that the clients dropped out of their rehabilitation program before it was finished. There was only one client who completed his rehabilitation plan and was unable to find work. Those who were successful in obtaining employment had vocational objectives in the professional/engineering or clerical/sales categories. Furthermore, 25 percent of those who dropped out of rehabilitation had no vocational objective formulated at the time of closure.

These data provide some baseline information on rehabilitation prior to the Rehabilitation Act of 1973, which gives top priority to those with severe disabilities. It will be interesting to see what impact this legislation has on such outcomes. However, these data are based on a highly selected group of persons. That is, using the standards of the late 1960s and early 1970s, which were harsher than today, the sample of 117 were admitted into rehabilitation because the probability of success (employment) was considered to be fairly high. Even so, 52 percent did not succeed. And if this group of 117 represented the *crème de la crème* in California at that time, how can we account for so many failures?

Rusk (1963) reported the results of a project to give specialized services to quadriplegics and noted that 23 of 25 persons with quadriplegia were placed in gainful employment. It is not known, however, if this definition of employment is the same as that currently used by state departments of rehabilitation or how long the persons held the job. To be placed in a job and to keep a job may be different.

However, Kaplan, Powell, Grynbaum, and Rusk (1966) and Dvonch, Kaplan, Grynbaum, and Rusk (1965) report data from a three-year follow-up on a group of 104 persons with spinal cord dysfunction. Fifty-three percent of this group was employed at some time since the onset of the disability. There are no data comparing the employed group with the unemployed group, and the group of 55 subjects contained only 13 persons with traumatic spinal injuries. Included in this group of 55 were 5 persons with multiple sclerosis and 2 with central nervous system syphilis; both progressive diseases may include intellectual impairments at some point.

However, keeping these complications in mind, these authors report that more education was indeed associated with employment. In comparing those still employed at follow-up with those who had been employed at some time since onset but not at the time of the follow-up, the former group had a 10 percent higher average salary prior to disability and a 32 percent higher salary during postdisability employment. In addition, the former group showed a more stable work picture both prior to and after disability, had a higher proportion of persons who drove their own car to work, and were an average of 5.9 years younger than the no-longer employed group. We do not know if employment in this study included full-time and part-time work, and in-home or outside employment; however, 55 percent of this study group of 55 cases were currently employed at follow-up, which is 29 percent of the total group of 104 who had been discharged from the New York University Medical Center.

Siegel (1969a, 1969b, 1971), from the same institution, reported follow-up studies of persons with quadriplegia, one of which seems to be the group described by Rusk (1963). They sent postcards of inquiry to 355 persons with quadriplegia who had been hospitalized between 1948 and 1960. It is not known if quadriplegia was defined in the same broad manner as Dvonch et al. (1965) and Kaplan et al. (1966), but this probably is the case since these studies all emanated from the same institution. Therefore, it must be assumed that these data include other than traumatic spinal injury. Of the total group of 355 persons, 177 replied to the postcard which asked about employment status. Thirty-nine percent of the 177 responded that they were employed; 10 percent were in college. However, if the total group of 355 is used and if those who did not respond are presumed to be unemployed (a questionable assumption), then, at worst, the figure is 19 percent employment. Another follow-up of persons with quadriplegia had a sample of 131 persons who had been hospitalized between 1962 and 1967. Thirty-four percent were in competitive employment, 2 percent were homemakers, and 47 percent were in college or special vocational training programs. Since the experience had been that those who successfully complete a college education have good prospects for competitive employment, Siegel expressed optimism about the total success rate for those in his study. These are among the most promising figures reported but unfortunately the outcome of this group is not known. Siegel (1970) does emphasize, however, the importance of independent means of transportation in obtaining and maintaining employment.

Rosenthal (1966) followed 32 persons with traumatic spinal injury who had been hospitalized at his institution. Out of the 24 who were considered capable of going to school or work, only 1 was gainfully employed and 4 were attending school. Unfortunately, there is little information about the nature of his sample of persons.

Felton and Litman (1965) evaluated 222 men with ''spinal cord injury'' who responded to a questionnaire about successful occupational adjustment, defined as employed in an area commensurate with one's training. The authors caution that interpretation of their data is tentative because of the self-selection by the respondents. Furthermore, the size of the original sample is not known. Eighty-five percent of the respondents were veterans, and combat injuries accounted for the largest number of injuries. Twenty-four percent of the group were disabled from various diseases. Of the total group, 58 percent were employed, 30 percent were unemployed, and 10 percent were in school. Of those persons with paraplegia, 60 percent were employed. For persons with quadriplegia, the employment figure was 48 percent. The authors state:

> The high proportion of employed quadriplegic men in the present sample may be accounted for by the voluntary character of the sample as a whole, and the fact that many subjects belonged to organizations of disabled persons with strong motivations for rebuilding their lives. (Felton and Litman 1965, p. 810)

In addition, they found that the unemployed had the lowest educational level and the smallest mean difference in predisability and postdisability education. In seeking jobs, persons with quadriplegia experienced the greatest number of job rejections of those who were employed. The unemployed had the fewest number of job rejections thus raising the question as to whether they had used less effort to obtain employment. Among the employed, 48 percent had received vocational training, whereas only 27 percent of the unemployed had such training; however, few of the respondents were working in jobs for which they were trained. Thus, the authors conclude that vocational training induces a sense of worth by teaching persons with spinal injury that they do have skills and abilities. Level of disability was not related to number currently employed, but it was related to number of job rejections.

Geisler, Jousse, and Wynne-Jones (1966a and 1966b) studied 1,204 persons with paraplegia or quadriplegia from disease or injury in Canada. Of this group, 46 percent were employed and 5 percent were in school or training. Employment according to level of completeness of injury was 25 percent for complete quadriplegia, 38 percent for partial quadriplegia, and 50 percent for paraplegia. Becoming disabled prior to age 40 and more education were associated with higher employment rates. This was particularly true for complete quadriplegics.

Wilson (1972) sent a postcard to each of 206 persons with quadriplegia of traumatic etiology who had participated in the rehabilitation program at his vocational rehabilitation center from January 1959 through May 1969. Of those postcards sent, 97 were returned with usable information. There were 91 males and 6 females. For the 91 males, there were 140 admissions to the center suggesting that rehabilitation was a multistage process and required considerable time for some persons. Forty-five persons with quadriplegia completed their vocational training program, and 40 percent of these persons, or 18, were employed after receiving vocational training. Forty-four percent of the total group of 97 eventually found employment. Including those who were in school, 49 percent of the total group were involved in school or work. These data are comparable to those reported by Brown and Chanin (1974) and Chanin and Brown (1975) in that both report success at achieving employment following training programs sponsored by state departments of rehabilitation. Both groups were composed of individuals who were considered feasible for employment and who had received some advanced training. Therefore, there must be some other significant factors reducing the employment rate of such promising groups.

Seybold (1976) reports data on a group of non-service-connected disabilities in veterans receiving a small pension that is reduced once they obtain independent income. In a survey sponsored by the Paralyzed Veterans of America, only 13 percent of these men were employed. The reasons given for not working were: the disability was too severe (48 percent), and they would lose more by working at full capacity than they now receive in benefits (28 percent).

Goldberg and Freed (1976) followed a group of persons with spinal injury and found that 14 percent were employed in the competitive labor market, 34 percent were involved in school activity or homemaking, and 52 percent were unemployed.

These studies suggest that between 13 percent and 48 percent of persons with spinal injury become involved in competitive employment. However, it is difficult to compare these studies because the subject population varies in terms of self-selection, the amount of vocational training, the time since onset of injury, and the age range. Employment may be defined in various ways, and number of hours worked is not known in most cases. Essentially, these data suggest that if success is defined as employment, then we have not been very successful. However, employment may not be an appropriate goal for all persons; many persons who would like to work cannot find a job, and some people who would like to work, cannot afford to take a job. Therefore, more of the variables associated with obtaining employment must be explored.

VARIABLES ASSOCIATED WITH EMPLOYMENT

At what point following spinal injury should the topic of work be introduced? Professionals tend to enjoy their jobs and forget that a significant proportion of the labor force in the United States does not enjoy work because it is monotonous and unrewarding to them (Terkel 1972, 1974). In addition, Caywood (1974) describes his rejection of any discussion of vocational endeavors when he got to the rehabilitation center. He was so busy learning to cope with his physical world that his future job was the least of his worries at that time.

There are two schools of thought on the issue of timing regarding vocational matters. Some believe that the entire team, including the rehabilitation counselor, should become involved with the person soon after injury. The degree of involvement by the rehabilitation counselor at this point is a question to be researched. Others believe that the process of rehabilitation takes a very long time and that it is premature to discuss vocational matters very early after injury. O'Connor and Leitner (1971) believe that the optimum time for reemployment is two to three years after injury. However, Carter (1977) believes that the person needs two years just to become comfortable with the physical and social changes spinal injury entails. After two years or so, depending on the individual, the person will be more able to incorporate the demands of schooling, vocational training, or employment. Kerr and Thompson (1972) also believe that it takes at least two years for the mental adjustment process to be completed. Thus, a question for research is the timing of vocational efforts. Are persons with spinal injury more likely to participate in and complete a training program two or three years after injury versus one year after injury? Do the employment rates differ according to this timing?

Studies reviewed in previous sections of this chapter indicate that a college education, predisability employment stability, and ability to drive a car were associated with employment following spinal injury, along with other variables. To assess the process of making vocational plans, Goldberg and Freed (1973) studied 21 persons who were approximately one year postinjury and rated them on their degree of involvement in vocational planning before and after the disability. They found that the group as a whole tended to lower their educational plans, vocational plans, and reasons for work interests following disability. However, they found that acceptance of responsibility for vocational plans prior to disability was the most frequent predictor of vocational planning. Work interests prior to disability were the next most frequent predictor of postdisability vocational planning. Persons with more work-related interests were more motivated to obtain or return to work. Those who accepted responsibility for predisability educational plans were more likely to find work intrinsically satisfying. Interestingly, persons with less severe disabilities tended to be more realistic in their interests, whereas persons with complete quadriplegia either tended to have more fantasies about what they could do or had reduced their interests following disability. Also, age was a predictor of postdisability vocational planning. Older persons were more realistic as to what a job required and their ability to do a job than were younger persons. Younger persons seemed more overwhelmed by the disability and concentrated on survival, whereas older persons were a bit more optimistic in their outlook. In fact, the older person's remotivation to return to work was greater than the younger person's desire to obtain work. Thus, previous experience with the world of work and education were definite assets following spinal injury.

Four years later, Goldberg and Freed (1976) followed up this sample to assess outcome. As reported earlier, 14 percent were employed and 34 percent were in school or homemaking. In addition, they found that those who had formulated concrete plans to accomplish a vocational objective tended to obtain full-time employment or to be enrolled in school full time. Those who derived intrinsic satisfaction from work spent more time in the competitive labor market than those whose interests were extrinsic to the job. Persons who had formulated educational plans that were concrete, specific, and related to vocational goals had less difficulties in obtaining work after discharge. Those with less severe disabilities were more optimistic and had a greater motivation to return to work consistent with their abilities and interests. However, severity of disability per se was not associated with productivity later. Timing was an issue. Those who had experienced the disability for a longer period of time had higher work values; that is, work was more important to them. And, as found in other studies, preinjury level of education was associated with postdisability employment. Other predictors of employment were the responsibility for a large number of children, more school training, and fewer functional limitations. Marital status per se was not associated with employment.

These authors interpret their data as reflecting the process of vocational development, which occurs along a continuum from birth to death, and view spinal injury as constituting an episode in one's life. As a result of spinal injury, vocational development does not cease. Rather, it is interrupted while the person learns to adapt to the changes in life. Then the vocational development picks up where it had temporarily stopped. Therefore, they recommend that vocational counselors should focus on the person's predisability development as a basis for making postdisability plans. This approach seems most consistent with the data reviewed in this document.

Kemp and Vash (1971) in a sample of 50 cases found that productivity (defined as various activities in addition to employment), at least five years after spinal cord injury, was associated with having a large number of family, work, or avocationally oriented goals. In addition, the most productive persons expressed their greatest loss in activity rather than physical terms and were more creative in problem solving. Interpersonal support was a significant factor for persons with quadriplegia but not for paraplegia. Level of injury per se was not associated with productivity, nor was preinjury level of employment or education.

El Ghatit and Hanson (1978) report that male spinal injured veterans who were most likely to have obtained employment included those: injured prior to age 30, injured for at least five years, paraplegic rather than quadriplegic, married, educated and trained beyond high school, able to drive an automobile, and able to care for own bladder and bowel. Of course, some persons not meeting these qualifications did find work. The best predictor of obtaining employment was simply whether or not the person had actively sought employment.

Thus, it would seem that given the present system, some persons have a greater probability of becoming employed following spinal injury than others. Essentially, those persons with some educational or vocational accomplishments prior to injury tend to continue this pattern after injury. However, a core issue in this regard may be the internal versus external locus of control dimension which was discussed in chapter 3. Is it possible that those who perceive their own behavior as controlling most of the rewards of the world are the ones who have accepted responsibility for educational and vocational planning prior to disability and who then continue this pattern after disability, as Goldberg and Freed (1973, 1976) found? Do the externals remain more overwhelmed by the disability and either fail to initiate a vocational training program or fail to finish such a program? Do externals seek fewer jobs and fail to persist in the face of employer rejections?

Felton (1964) studied the attitudes of employers toward hiring the disabled and found that those who had had experience with disabled employees were least restrictive in their perceptions about what disabled persons could or could not do. The major reasons for not hiring the handicapped cited by employers who were not knowledgeable about disability were lack of mobility and manipulative skills, problems created by physical arrangement of the plant or office, the (presumed) characteristic personality attributes of the disabled, and the reaction of others to the disability. Infrequently cited, but present, were such factors as insurance restrictions, accident or injury risks, and the handicapped worker's difficulty in gaining sufficient work experience.

The reasons for rejection given to the disabled person by the employer were insurance company regulations or physical inaccessibility of the job setting; yet, in actuality, the employers believed that disabled persons were only suitable for jobs that could be done independently and in isolation, and they were very skeptical about any job in which the disabled person was expected to exercise authority over coworkers or function in a professional status. In addition, the employers preferred to minimize any interactions between the disabled person and the public. Thus, another factor in the statistics on employment of persons with spinal injury is the negative and unrealistic perception employers have regarding jobs suitable for the disabled. Persons with spinal injury generally obtain training and education in the professional/engineering or clerical/sales areas—the precise areas in which employers resist hiring. These jobs entail interactions with other employees and the public, the big concern of employers.

There is an additional factor that influences the statistics on employment of those with spinal injury: the financial disincentives to productivity. It should be recalled that Seybold (1976) found that 28 percent of non-service-connected veterans claimed that by going to work they would earn less than their veterans benefits paid them, and, therefore, they remained unemployed. Forty-eight percent of those unemployed claimed that their disability was too severe for them to be able to work; however, in actuality, many people who are very severely disabled do indeed work. Thus, one wonders if these persons were also influenced by the financial disincentives of returning to work, but did not admit it. There is heavy pressure on every man in the United States to be gainfully employed unless he has a legitimate excuse. We do not know how many persons with severe disabilities would willingly become involved in employment efforts (assuming a more receptive attitude by employers) if they were not penalized financially.

Deyoe (1972b) studied 242 veterans with spinal injury and found that 62, or 26 percent, were employed either full or part time, either in or out of their homes. Of these, only 7 non-service-connected veterans had found full-time employment with sufficient income to preclude their veterans pension or social security payments. Deyoe states:

> Therefore, it may be concluded that a veteran with service-connected disability often can afford not to work, while a veteran with nonservice-connected disability as often cannot afford to work. (Deyoe 1972b, p. 528)

A service-connected veteran is one whose disability was sustained while in the service. For most persons with paraplegia and quadriplegia, the yearly benefit, tax free, approaches $20,000 as of 1979. In addition, the person is eligible for care at the Veterans Administration hospitals at no cost. No matter what other income the person has, he never loses these benefits.

For the non-service-connected veteran, the situation is very different. This person sustained his disability while out of the service, but may be eligible for a veterans pension. The maximum monthly pension for him is $340.00, or $4,080.00 a year, as of October 1977. For each $2.00 of income he receives, he loses $1.00 of his pension. When his income exceeds $4,100.00 a year, he loses all veterans pension and the right to ambulatory care at the Veterans Administration hospitals. He remains eligible for inpatient care, but priority is given to the needs of service-connected veterans in terms of admissions.

The requirements for Social Security Disability Income (SSDI) and Supplemental Security Income (SSI) state that anyone able to earn $240.00 per month, defined as substantial gainful activity (SGA), is not disabled, *regardless of the degree of physical disability present.* When the person earns more than this amount, he or she loses the SSDI and SSI benefits and loses eligibility for Medicaid or Homemaker/Chore services. However, *the costs of survival for the disabled are significantly greater than for the nondisabled person,* and, therefore, disabled persons require a very high salary from employment efforts in order to be able to afford to give up the various benefits to which they are entitled.

For example, Tanaka (1977) points out that transportation is a requirement for gainful employment out of the house. Yet public transportation is inaccessible, and the person must own a car that has automatic transmission, hand controls, and that is large enough to accommodate a wheelchair easily. This eliminates the small, economically priced car and usually means that the car belongs to the category, "gas guzzler," which is an additional expense. Inability to use self-service gasoline increases the cost of transportation as does the requirement that all service and maintenance must be purchased. The cost of a van is even greater. A wheelchair accessible home may cost more, especially if modifications must be made. Assistance with cleaning, cooking, and laundry may be necessary which means hiring someone to help. Wheelchairs cost money, require repair and replacement, and the appliances associated with bladder and bowel management, along with medications, all cost money. Thus, the basics of survival as a disabled person require more money than for a nondisabled person.

Going to work usually means the loss of Medicaid benefits, and private insurance is prohibitively expensive. Thus, persons with disabilities must work for an organization that provides group health insurance benefits, but the provisions of these policies usually exclude any expenses that are related to the disability.

Given the attitudinal barriers of employers and the costs of living with a disability, we can understand the data on gainful full-time employment among persons with spinal injury. There are many legitimate costs to a disability that cannot be met without a high salary. In addition, acceptance of a job and elimination of the SSDI, SSI, or veterans pension means that the person loses medical coverage for matters associated with the disability. Many decide that they cannot take that risk. Thus, we have a twofold problem: a survival level income and medical coverage. This becomes another "Catch 22." Society defines employment as a key criterion of acceptance, and all rehabilitation efforts have been aimed at full-time employment, but most persons with disabilities cannot afford to take a job.

The Comprehensive Service Needs Study (1975) recommends a separation of the income maintenance and health care coverage provisions of current welfare legislation. The report suggests that health care coverage be extended to all severely disabled persons regardless of employment or income, but with reasonable cost-sharing provisions. Furthermore, the recommendation was made to expand the scope of services covered to include equipment maintenance and repair, and attendant care. They conclude:

> Many programs contain severe disincentives to the vocational rehabilitation of the severely handicapped because the programs are predicated on assumptions of labor force retirement (not employed). Since these income maintenance programs bestow needed cash on the severely handicapped, usually have concomitant medical benefits, and open eligibility to other programs as well, the cumulative benefits often require very high wage options before persons have incentives to show they are capable of labor force participation. We do not

suggest persons are malingering, but that motivation is often necessary to overcome a handicap and without it, persons will not strive. Legislative changes would be required to allow these programs to be based on severity alone and not on labor force withdrawal, so that the severely handicapped would work without significant penalties in lost benefits. (Executive Summary of Comprehensive Service Needs Study 1975, p. 23)

Consequently, there are several variables associated with employment of persons with spinal injury: timing of the vocational program; intrinsic characteristics of the person; employer attitudes and discrimination; the financial disincentives to productivity; and the procedures we use to assist the person in achieving a vocational objective. This latter issue should be examined more closely.

STRATEGIES OF VOCATIONAL REHABILITATION

It seems that much of the literature has focused on statements that persons with spinal injury can work and on the identification of those factors within the person that predict success or failure in employment. However, as noted above, there are many environmental variables that influence the employment rate, yet little research effort has been directed at the identification of these environmental factors and methods of modifying their effects. One of these environmental variables that must be considered and that has not been studied definitively is the operational policy of departments of rehabilitation. Walker (1961) stated years ago that,

In reality, the inabilities of patients to achieve appropriate goals do not represent failures by the patient, but by rehabilitation personnel who have not developed techniques and programs which tap patient resources. . . . Until we are able to improve the quality of programs in the psychologic, social, and vocational areas as well as medical, the percentage of quadriplegics who become employed will continue to remain low. (Walker 1961, pp. 720-21)

Have we made great advances in developing techniques and programs that tap patient resources? Little and Stewart (1975) do not believe so. There are some isolated examples of intensive efforts to evaluate the person, train the person, and place the person, as described by Siegel (1969a), but these efforts are not the customary procedure across the United States. Within vocational rehabilitation, we have persisted in assuming that the only factor leading to success will be the intrinsic characteristics and abilities of the client, and the role of the environment continues to be ignored. Because of this assumption, there has been little effort devoted to the development of strategies to identify the strengths of each individual, develop these strengths, and then place the person in a job that he or she can perform. We have focused almost exclusively on college education or training for professional/engineering or clerical/sales jobs. Are there no other jobs that a person with spinal injury can perform? What happens to the people who do not have the talent or ability for these kinds of jobs? Must they be excluded from the world of work? How do we evaluate candidates for vocational rehabilitation? Do we rely exclusively on psychological tests or do we use work samples? Poor (1975) and Poor, Fletcher, Thielges, Gutknecht, and Morgan (1975) have described some of the various evaluation procedures possible. Crewe, Athelstan, and Meadows (1975) discuss the necessity of making vocational diagnoses through an assessment of functional limitations, rather than by use of medical or psychiatric diagnoses. However, we still have theories of career development being propounded that emphasize the stages of adjustment in psychodynamic terms and that implicitly place all of the responsibility for vocational success on the shoulders of the person with spinal injury (Schlenoff 1975). As long as rehabilitation counselors utilize such theories as an approach to their clients, we will not improve our success rate regarding employment of persons with spinal injury. This has been the predominant emphasis in theory and in practice, and it has not worked.

Crewe, Athelstan, and Bower (1978) have made an admirable attempt to fill this void by publishing a handbook for vocational counselors documenting the postinjury work experiences of 100 persons with spinal injury. Their intent is to generate new ideas about the employment options of persons with paraplegia and quadriplegia. In addition to biographies of these 100 persons, Crewe and her associates discuss the role of employment within the overall rehabilitation of persons with spinal injury and provide information and suggestions that should be helpful to vocational counselors in their work with severely disabled persons.

Thus, we need to consider *each* person to be a candidate for some job, and we must assess the person's strengths using multiple evaluation strategies, psychological tests, and behavior samples. We must develop procedures to translate these strengths into usable skills, employing behavioral principles since this is a learning process (Karan and Gardner 1973). We need to have job placement specialists within each rehabilitation agency whose task is to identify jobs in the community and to place the person in the job most suitable for him or her.

Although these efforts may be helpful and are needed improvements over our current procedures, by themselves they will not influence the employment rate significantly unless the financial disincentives to productivity are removed. Therefore, if employment is a goal, and if each person with spinal injury shall have the option of gainful employment, we need to focus our efforts in two directions simultaneously. We need to develop techniques for increasing the skills of persons with spinal injury, and we need to demonstrate that the removal of the financial disincentives in our social legislation will lead to increased productivity. The elimination of these financial disincentives will require the *recognition that the costs of living at a survival level are greater for the disabled person than for the able-bodied person.* Thus, some amount of guaranteed annual income, plus access to low-cost medical treatment, may be necessary and these should not be reduced no matter what the person earns. As a result, employment could be financially rewarding, as well as intrinsically rewarding, to the person who chooses to owrk.

Removal of the financial disincentives to productivity will not lead to the employment of everyone with a disability. Employment may not be an appropriate goal for everyone, and there are many parameters to productivity. However, there are a large number of persons with disabilities who have the desire to work and the skills necessary to get a job, but they cannot take the financial risks of giving up the minimal benefits they do have. If these people were able to obtain employment without financially penalizing themselves, the statistics on employment rate would improve significantly. Furthermore, if these individuals were assisted in the placement process by departments of rehabilitation, the employment rate would improve.

Therefore, a research project should be funded that would remove the financial disincentives from a large sample of people who were also given evaluation, training, and placement services by departments of rehabilitation. This sample must be large and representative of the United States population of persons with spinal injury. The study should be funded for several years, perhaps five years, in order to provide an adequate test of the question. As a result of this project, more realistic figures on the employment potential of persons with spinal injury could be obtained.

VOLUNTARISM

There are many parameters to productivity, and employment is only one. Membership in groups, participation in community organizations, and volunteering of services are viable activities that may supplement or substitute for employment activities, depending upon the person. With increasing numbers of mothers of small children entering the labor force, daycare centers have developed around the United States. Since staffing is often a problem, the use of physically disabled volunteers could accomplish two goals: provide a sense of purpose to the life of the disabled person and educate young children about the abilities of persons with physical disabilities. The use of physically disabled vounteers in schools, hospitals, rehabilitation centers, and other areas could accomplish the same two goals. Thus, greater attention should be given to this parameter of daily life among disabled persons.

SUMMARY

The literature is replete with articles demonstrating that persons with spinal injury can be employed, and most of the research has focused on the identification of the characteristics of the person who succeeds in obtaining gainful employment. This research suggests that previous education and employment may be predictive of reemployment after disability but may not be correlated with overall productivity. A preinjury pattern of accepting responsibility for educational and vocational planning portends well for the person's future after injury. Being creative in problem solving, having many goals, focusing on activity versus physical function, and having interpersonal support have been found to be associated with productivity. But, productivity encompasses more than employment, and employment may not be an appropriate goal for all persons with disabilities.

The literature focuses almost exclusively on the person variables related to employment, but little attention has been given to environmental variables such as employer attitudes and discrimination, the financial disincentives to productivity, and the procedures of departments of rehabilitation.

Recent HEW regulations are aimed at removing discrimination by employers. Yet without a removal of the financial disincentives to productivity, the statistics on employment will remain relatively static. Furthermore, emphasis needs to be placed on the development of strategies to identify a person's strengths, to train these strengths into marketable skills, and to place the person in a suitable job rather than relying exclusively on college education for a career in the professions. A variety of jobs need to be identified so that each person with a disability can have the option of gainful employment.

6
Sexuality and Spinal Cord Injury

The issue of sexuality and spinal cord injury overlaps significantly with the three previous chapters; it is being treated here as a separate issue only for the purposes of organization. Most of the issues considered in the chapter on the psychological variables will influence one's sexuality, and certainly the social variables discussed in chapter 4 must be considered in any discussion of sexual behaviors. There is also considerable opinion that a satisfactory sexual life is correlated with productivity.

In earlier papers, Trieschmann (1973) and Griffith, Trieschmann, Hohmann, Cole, Tobis, and Cummings (1975) have emphasized the necessity of differentiating among sex drive, sex acts, and sexuality when dealing with a person with a physical disability.

Sex is a primary drive, as are hunger, thirst, and avoidance of pain, to name several. These primary drives are expressed through the complex interrelationship of bodily receptors, hormonal balance, the autonomic nervous system, and the central nervous system. Ordinarily, the potential for expression of the sex drive is present from birth to death, but certain situations may interfere with the ability to express this drive. Both men and women may find that malaise, pain, or daily nervous tension may interfere with the sex drive on any one occasion. Unfortunately, the onset of chronic illness or physical disability was assumed to eliminate sex drives, and, for many years, this assumption governed the behavior of rehabilitation and health care professionals. However, in the last decade this assumption has been challenged and sexual functioning is being introduced as a legitimate part of rehabilitation programs. Therefore, in considering the rehabilitation of persons with spinal injury, the issue of sex drives must be examined.

Sex acts are those behaviors involving the erogenous zones and genital areas that may, but need not, include sexual intercourse. There are an infinite variety of sex acts that involve motor behavior and that produce a pleasurable sensory response. Many areas of the body may participate in this sensory sexual response, the genital area being a primary but not exclusive one. Through sex acts, we express our sex drive, but learning plays a significant role in determining which sex acts a person considers to be permissible and whom the appropriate partners are (Ford and Beach 1951). Thus, following spinal injury, certain kinds of sex acts may become difficult or impossible, especially in men, and, consequently, the issue of the variety of sex acts considered to be permissible by a disabled person becomes a critical issue (Mooney, Cole, and Chilgren 1975).

Yet the sex drive and various sex acts cannot become the focus of rehabilitation without considering the issue of sexuality. Sexuality is the expression of a sex drive, through sex acts, within the context of the sexual identity of the person: the maleness and femaleness of the individual which is so heavily influenced by learning and one's environment. In describing female sexuality, Romano (1973a) states:

> Sexuality is more than the act of sexual intercourse. It involves for most women the whole business of relating to another person: the tenderness, the desire to give as well as take, the compliments, casual caresses, reciprocal concerns, tolerance, the forms of communication that both include and go beyond words. For women, sexuality includes a range of behaviors from smiling through orgasm; it is not just what happens between two people in bed. (Romano 1973a, p. 28)

This concept of sexuality may apply to men also, but not one description of this kind about men could be found in the literature on sex and physical disability. Admittedly, a certain proportion of men do view sex as the act of sexual intercourse which provides them with a feeling of physical release and masculine validation. But many men find sex acts infinitely more rewarding within the context of a good relationship. Perhaps men do not feel as free to describe this in the literature as do women. Nichols (1975) in his book about men's liberation points out that men may profit from a cultural revolution in order to develop all sides of their personality, just as women have in recent years. It is interesting to note the number of articles in the literature that label a section, sexuality, and then proceed to discuss genital function only.

It is a thesis of this chapter that sexual rehabilitation of the person with spinal injury requires that the person be evaluated in terms of his or her sex drive, his or her preferred sex acts, and his or her sexuality. A lack of differentiation among these concepts and a general reference to sexual function alone may lead to an evaluation that does not clearly identify the important parameters of the problem. Only through careful evaluation of these three issues can we devise a treatment program specifically oriented to solving the problem. In addition, we will have a focus for research. Which techniques are successful in treating which aspects of a sexual dysfunction?

Griffith and Trieschmann (1976) propose that sexual dysfunctions in persons with physical disabilities usually have two components: a primary and a secondary component. Both must be evaluated and treated. Primary dysfunctions have organic impairments (neurological, endocrinological, urological, gynecological, musculo-skeletal, etc.) as their etiological base. Secondary dysfunctions are those in which there is no evidence of organic impairment to account for the difficulty. Rather, attitudes and anxieties interfere with sexual satisfaction, and the etiology is a behavioral one. Individuals with complete spinal cord injuries will have a primary sexual dysfunction, and probably a secondary sexual dysfunction as well, since spinal injury challenges not only physical capability but self-image and the concept of sexuality. Both dysfunctions must be evaluated and treated by a team of professionals who have knowledge about the physical and behavioral parameters of the case. Usually this entails a team composed of a physician and a psychologist or other professional with expertise in a variety of behavioral methods.

Thus, within both of these conceptual frameworks, there exist three components to sexual function: sex drive, sex acts, and sexuality. Each of these components may have a primary dysfunction and a secondary dysfunction, an organic problem and a behavioral problem. The remainder of this chapter will utilize these conceptual frameworks as an approach to the issue of sexual functioning following spinal injury.

SEXUAL FUNCTION AFTER SPINAL CORD INJURY

Sex Drives

In the last decade, the field of rehabilitation has discovered sex and attempts are being made to remedy the neglect of this issue in prior years. There was a time when a person with spinal injury was told that he would never marry, never have a family, and that he should put these issues out of his mind (Professional Conference 1977). This very devastating view of the world disappeared as advances in medical management changed the prognosis for those with spinal injury from grim to very good. However, the issue of sex was generally not mentioned by the rehabilitation staff, and patients did not raise the issue either in the 1950s and 1960s (Weiss and Diamond 1966). In the late 1960s and early 1970s, programs designed to reintroduce sexual function into rehabilitation were formulated (Romano and Lassiter 1972; Cole, Chilgren, and Rosenberg 1973); then the pendulum swing occurred from the belief that sex was not important following disability to the belief that sex was very important following spinal cord injury.

However, Hanson and Franklin (1976) asked 54 men with paraplegia and 74 men with quadriplegia to rank order the importance of various functions to them. First choice received a 1, second choice received a 2, etc. For persons with paraplegia, use of legs obtained a mean rank of 1.63, control of bladder and bowel ranked 1.83, and normal feeling and use of sex organs ranked 2.53. For persons with quadriplegia, the average rankings were use of arms and hands, 1.31; normal bladder and bowel function, 2.5; legs, 2.65; and sex,

3.54. Time since injury and marital status were not a factor in these ratings.

The rehabilitation staff rated how they expected persons with spinal injury to rank these functions. The mean ranks for the staff were: arms and hands, 1.62; sex, 2.5; bowel and bladder function, 2.69; and legs, 3.2. Hanson and Franklin conclude that the notion that sex is frequently the most devastating of all functional losses to men with spinal injury was not supported by the data. Two-thirds of the men ranked sex last in order of importance to them. But rehabilitation staff consistently overestimated the importance of sexual function to their patients.

Talbot (1971) believes that despite the physical impairment, the psychosexual content of ideation remains the same.

Allowing for the distractions of illness, discomfort, and fear, which are antagonistic to libidinous impulses in neurologically intact individuals as well, these patients retain the same erotic interests they exhibited before injury (Talbot 1971, p. 38)

But Hohmann's (1966) study on the experience of emotional feelings following spinal injury suggests that this may not be the case. This study was described in chapter 3. Four out of five persons in his cervical lesion group reported a marked decrease in feelings of sexual excitement, whereas one reported some decrease. They stated that satisfaction derived from pleasing a partner about whom they cared, but sex without a caring relationship was not rewarding. "It is a mental, thinking kind of thing rather than a physically driven feeling" (Hohmann 1966, p. 149). In the high thoracic group, four out of five reported a marked decrease in sexual feelings, and one reported some decrease. They described a mental interest in satisfying a close partner, and two reported some pleasant sensations from secondary erogenous zones. The low thoracic group reported some decrease in sexual feelings, and only one reported a marked decrease. Secondary erogenous zones were important sources of pleasant stimulation in this group, and two reported particular pleasure derived from a spot in the center of the back, just above the existing effective sensory level.

The lumbar group had one man who reported a marked decrease, and four reported some decrease in feelings of sexual excitement. They reported less tension and pressure for sex, and those with some psychogenic sexual function experienced an orgasm that was less exciting than before the injury. They called it a "paraorgasm." The sacral group had four who reported some decrease in sexual excitement and one reported no change. This group reported more drive for sexual activity than the other groups but felt more frustrated with such activity than any of the other groups.

Hohmann interpreted his results as being consistent with disruption of the autonomic nervous system which is associated with a generalized reduction in emotional feelings. He believes that there is some reduction in the sex drive following spinal injury and that presence of a partner with whom a good relationship exists becomes a critical issue in the maintenance of sexual activity after injury. Furthermore, he has observed that frequency of sexual activity within good marriages of 20–30 years duration tends to taper off at a more rapid rate than for nondisabled men in a similar age range (Hohmann 1977).

As mentioned in chapter 3, some persons with spinal injury contest Hohmann's findings of reduced emotional feelings since the injury. In regards to sexuality, they agree that a partner about whom they care is very important but emphasize that even before their injuries, a sexual relationship consisted of more than merely a genital response. They believe that there has been no change in this regard. Yet Hohmann, who has a spinal injury himself, can provide the reports of persons with spinal injury who perceive a reduction in experienced emotionality and a change in their experienced sex drive. Thus, this issue will require much more research before it is resolved.

Money (1960a) provides some corroboration for both the positions of Talbot and Hohmann. He found that sexual imagery and dreams did not change significantly from prior to injury. Those women who had many dreams of sexual activity prior to injury continued to do so after injury. Those who did not have such dreams preinjury did not have any of that kind after injury. Women who enjoyed sex prior to injury reported little satisfaction after injury, but they were willing to please a partner. However, there were only a few women in his sample.

For men, Money found a higher frequency of daydreams and night dreams about sex after injury than the women reported, but, as Hohmann described, the men reported sexual activity only if there was a close partner.

> Sex was a matter of memory, regretfully unobtainable, but not frantically striven for with desperate urgency. . . . Those patients who tried to have intercourse did so not for the erotic pleasure they themselves received, for there was none. Sexual desire was not experienced by these paraplegic patients as it was before injury, and they had no genitopelvic gratification. It is therefore all the more remarkable a phenomenon that some of them had orgasm imagery in dreams almost as vividly as though it were the real thing. (Money 1960a, pp. 380-381)

The phenomenon of phantom orgasm has been reported by a number of persons with spinal injury. They describe a buildup of tension with pleasurable sensations (although not genital sensations) which may be followed by a feeling of relaxation, perhaps with a temporary reduction of spasms. Comarr and Vigue (1978a, 1978b) report that ability to fantasize was related to ability to have an orgasm in a group of males and females with complete spinal injuries. However, they found that the females in their group far exceeded the males in ability to fantasize as a means of enhancing sexual pleasure. Thus, strategies to teach males to use fantasy became one focus for sexual counseling sessions. Money (1960b) discusses the cognitive components to eroticism, and Ford and Beach (1951) assert that the significance of the neocortical processes in sexual behavior increases greatly as one goes up the phylogenetic scale.

In order to summarize and integrate the above ideas, one might hypothesize that the experiences and behavioral repertoire that the person had prior to injury will have a great effect on function after injury. A man or woman who had positive and pleasurable sexual experiences prior to injury will approach sexual function after injury with a positive attitude if there is a partner present with whom he or she has a good relationship. There may be a decreased physical drive for sex, but pleasure may be obtained through satisfying a partner or by vicariously enjoying the partner's pleasure. In addition, the person may derive some pleasure from stimulation of secondary erogenous zones, such as the lips, neck, ears, nipples, and perhaps that segment of the body just above the level of the lesion. Certain individuals may be able to achieve a phantom orgasm if they had experienced orgasm prior to injury, and if they have a well-developed ability to fantasize. Individuals who do not have partners after injury but who had enjoyed sex prior to injury may daydream about sexual experiences but will not seek out partners for the purposes of sexual activity exclusively. One exception to this would be the experimentation that persons with spinal injury may seek soon after injury in order to test their ability to perform. Age of the person may be an important variable, with younger individuals retaining more of an interest in sexual activity than older persons. But this needs to be studied.

One would also hypothesize that individuals who were injured at an early age and who had limited sexual experience prior to injury would have more difficulty in initiating a relationship and becoming sexually involved with another person. Also one would predict that a person who had never experienced an orgasm prior to injury would have a low probability of experiencing a phantom orgasm after injury. However, these hypotheses must be tested through carefully controlled research.

Level of lesion may be a significant factor in interest in sexual activity. Hohmann (1966) found an inverse relationship between level of lesion and experience of emotional feelings. The higher the lesion, the less the intensity of emotions. Completeness of the lesion will certainly be a factor, since incomplete lesions allow for the possibility of intact pathways that relate cognitions of sexual stimuli to genital response.

Any differences between men and women with spinal injury reported in the literature may reflect cultural and generational influences. Traditionally, it was assumed that men had a greater sex drive than women, and women could get along without sexual satisfaction more easily than men. This assumption was probably transmitted to women who were born prior to 1950 and may have conditioned the responses that they give to researchers' questions. Many women raised in this sexually repressive climate learned that ''good'' women did not talk about sex and did not admit to a strong sex drive. Therefore, in any questionnaire and interview research on women with spinal injury, we must be aware of the possible discrepancy between what the woman says and what she does. Women born after 1950 may not be as guarded in discussing their sex lives, but ethnic, cultural, and social class variables may produce some inhibition.

Equally important to future research is the possible discrepancy between what the man with spinal injury says about his sex life and what he does. Men may feel that they must talk ''big'' about their sex lives in order to maintain their image as a man. Some men may feel somewhat embarrassed to admit that they desire sex less than they did preinjury and may attempt to conceal this with stories of their exploits.

Therefore, in assessing this issue of sex drive following spinal cord injury, it will be important to establish a close rapport with the subjects in order to ensure honesty of self-report. Age at the time of the study and age at onset may be important, as well as the presence of a partner with whom they have a good relationship. Thus, the issue of sex drive following spinal injury should be examined objectively. Does onset of spinal injury change one's sex drive? If we would discover that there is a reduction in sex drive, this would not eliminate the need for including sexual function in rehabilitation programs. Sexual function is one facet within social relationships, and every person with spinal cord inury should have the opportunity to learn to relate sexually to a partner if he or she chooses to do so.

Sex Acts Following Spinal Injury

There will be no attempt to describe the details of the physical impairments in sexual functioning following spinal injury, since there are several excellent reviews of the literature with extensive bibliographies. Griffith, Tomko, and Timms (1973) provide a comprehensive review of the factors associated with erection, ejaculation, and orgasm in men. In addition, Griffith, Timms, and Tomko (1972) have edited a series of abstracts of articles on this topic that provides more detail to supplement their review of the literature. Rabin (1974) has written a book for the person with spinal injury which documents these details also. Information on women is limited and the review of the literature by Griffith and Trieschmann (1975) should be consulted along with the article by Romano (1973a).

In essence, spinal cord injury produces an impairment in motor and sensory function. Genital sensation is lost in complete lesions, and erections occur by reflex and are not associated with psychosexual stimuli. The higher the lesion, the greater the role of reflex in erection. Lumbar lesions that are complete sometimes result in a flaccid penis, and reflex erections do not occur, whereas with sacral lesions that are complete, flaccidity is constant. With incomplete lesions, the probability of psychogenic erections increases, and erective capacity is usually not as impaired.

Ejaculation in complete lesions is usually impaired, and the seminal fluid is ejected into the bladder. not out of the urethra. Orgasm, in the physical sense, is not perceived and fertility in men is markedly impaired. With incomplete lesions, ejaculation and orgasm may not be impaired.

Therefore, men with spinal injury may be able to participate in sexual intercourse if they can obtain and sustain an erection long enough for the partner to reach orgasm. With strong upper extremity function and a lower level lesion, the man may be able to assume the superior position. However, the side-lying and female superior position are often used.

Female sexual function following spinal injury is frequently summed up with a terse statement about her relatively unimpaired sexual function because of her traditionally passive role in sex. Menstruation resumes within several months of injury, and her ability to conceive and bear children are relatively unimpaired. Therefore, Griffith and Trieschmann (1975) note that a review of the available information published in the literature might lead to the erroneous conclusion that women with spinal injuries have no sex drive, that they engage in only one sex act (intercourse in the supine position), and that their sexuality consists of the ability to conceive and deliver babies. Romano (1973a) presents a very eloquent and integrated view of sexual function focusing on the disabled woman's sexuality and the many kinds of sex acts that are expressions of the woman's sexuality.

Despite the loss of sensation and motor function following spinal injury, a woman's ability to participate in most sex acts seems to be unimpaired. The woman with a high cervical lesion will be passive in a motoric sense only and retains the ability to be very active in all of the interpersonal aspects of sexuality. Women with lesions in the low cervical, thoracic, and lumbosacral regions may remain active in various degrees of motor activity of a sexual nature and, of course, can be very active interpersonally. They can participate in all of the kinds of communication that are a part of a relationship between two caring people.

We do not know much about the woman's ability to lubricate the vaginal opening and vaginal wall prior to or during intercourse. Nor do we know if the physiological stages of sexual excitement, as described by Masters and Johnson (1966) in the able-bodied woman, occur reflexively in women with spinal injury. There are clinical reports of a sex flush and increased sensitivity of the nipple and breast regions in women who retain sensation in that area. There are also clinical reports of phantom orgasms in women who had preinjury sexual experiences that were positive and pleasurable.

If we are going to study sexual function in men and women with spinal injury, we must broaden our focus to include the multitude of sex acts that form a pattern of communication between two caring people, rather than persisting in focusing exclusively on sex acts that are motoric and genital. We must begin to view sexual function as encompassing more than sexual intercourse only.

Cole, Chilgren, and Rosenberg (1973) report that in their group of persons with spinal injury who attended a workshop, 45 percent had sexual intercourse less than once a month, in comparison to 12 percent of the able-bodied participants. More persons with paraplegia believed that a satisfactory sex life was important than persons with quadriplegia. In regards to oral-genital sexual activity, 90 percent of the persons with quadriplegia, in comparison to 60 percent of the persons with paraplegia, found the idea attractive, suggesting that sexual intercourse is not the exclusive issue in the lives of these persons.

Berkman, Weissman, and Frielich (1978) studied 145 male veterans with spinal injury. Most had partners. Of those who were sexually active, only 32 percent reported engaging in sexual intercourse every time they had sex relations, even though 70 percent reported that they had erections. In addition, 48 percent reported engaging in oral-genital activity and 25 percent used manual stimulation alone. Of those men who abstained from sexual activity, 40 percent were married. Lack of sexual experience after injury was not correlated with degree of adjustment to the disability. This substantiates Hohmann's (1972) contention that,

> A substantial number of marriages between cord injured men and their wives—based on a sexual relationship consisting of a profound love, affection, and understanding combined with only the most casual petting, kissing, and other expressions of tenderness—have continued with a good relationship for more than a quarter of a century. (Hohmann 1972, p. 54)

Sexuality

Berkman and associates (1978) define sexuality as a dynamic process based on developmental learning experiences having three components: the psychosexual component in which the individual's self-concept is central; the social sexual component which characterizes relations with others; and the behavioral component which focuses on specific sexual behaviors. They state that sexual development, like other forms of human growth, is an ongoing process in which new learning occurs throughout life. Sexual expressions may change, they go on to state, because of personal needs, interpersonal experiences, and as a result of physical limitations.

These authors present a theme that is consistent with that emphasized in this book. A person's life evolves as a result of many learning experiences, and spinal injury is one episode in this developmental process. Accommodations are made to the spinal injury consistent with the person's preinjury development and the spinal injury, while significant, may not be the most important event in the person's life.

The impact of spinal cord injury on a person's sexuality will be closely related to the impact on his self-concept, view of himself, self-esteem (Lovitt 1970; Crigler 1974; Schimel 1974; Singh and Magner 1975), and will be highly influenced by his skill and confidence in interpersonal relationships. Harlow (1971) describes the process of learning to love, based on his research with primates, which suggests that the basis for adult interpersonal and sexual relationships is learned at a very early age. This process of learning to love probably occurs in all humans, and, thus, the impact of spinal cord injury on sexuality will vary depending on how well one has learned to be able to love.

One's sexuality usually is not an issue in solitary situations. Rather, the concept of sexuality implies an interactive process with at least one other person. The various means of communication become the core issue of sexuality, and physical attractiveness may be a critical factor in initial contacts. In order to have the opportunity to communicate with another person, there has to be some way to arrange contact among strangers. And among strangers, physical attractiveness is an important variable in prompting initial contact and liking for a partner (Berscheid and Walster 1974). Many persons with spinal injury indicate that they take much greater care with their physical appearance following the injury, both men and women. One man described his greater interest in having a ''mod'' hairstyle and mustache and attractive clothing. One woman who had been a strong advocate of women's liberation prior to her injury began to wear a bra and try to appear more ''feminine'' following her injury (Consumer Conference 1977).

Bregman and Hadley (1976) describe the range of sexual behaviors among 31 women with spinal injury and report that sexual adjustment was not related to duration of the disability or to having received information about their sexual capabilities. The giving of information about their ability to have sexual intercourse, menstruation, and pregnancy did not assist the women in their sexual adjustment. Most of the women found that their first sexual experience after injury was psychologically uncomfortable because they feared rejection. This fear persisted for some time especially for divorced and single women. They found that as time provided them with more experience they gradually developed the courage to experiment, and sexual experiences became more positive.

In addition, Bregman and Hadley found that women who appeared to feel good about themselves psychologically also claimed to be adjusting well sexually. As they began to feel like themselves again, their social relationships began to improve, and their sexual relationships improved. Those who appeared to have poor self-images seemed to be having more difficulty adjusting sexually. The subjects stressed the importance of open and honest communication with their partners, and many of the women derived great sexual pleasure despite their impaired sensation and motor function. The authors conclude that the psychological aspects of sexuality are extremely important to sexual excitement, and they wonder if the psychological role is even more powerful than the physical one.

Fitting, Salisbury, Davies, and Mayclin (1978) found a positive relationship between a spinal injured woman's self-concept and her sexuality. The women in their study perceived themselves as more assertive, more independent, more active as a sexual partner, more intellectual, and more honest with themselves after injury than before injury. Although their images of themselves as women had changed since the spinal injury, many felt that the changes were related to maturation rather than to the spinal injury exclusively.

It is of interest to note that Berkman and associates (1978) found that only 41 percent of the males who were sexually active rated their sexual relations as satisfactory, although 76 percent believed that their partners were satisfied.

These authors found that higher sexual adjustment scores were correlated with younger age, injury at a younger age, higher level of income, better physical function, better performance in the roles of worker and community participant, higher morale, positive attitudes of self-acceptance, and independence. Duration of disability and marital status were not correlated with level of sexual adjustment. However, abstinence from sexual activity was not correlated with psychological, social, or physical measures of adjustment to disability. They conclude that absence of sexual activity may be one form of adjustment to life among the disabled and nondisabled alike.

This latter point should be emphasized. We may assume that adjustment to disability entails satisfactory sexual activity. This may not be the case. Sexual activity is one of the activities of life and not necessarily the most important one. We need to consider multiple parameters of adjustment, and sexual activity may not be necessary for satisfaction for everyone. It is interesting to note that the women studied by Bregman and Hadley seem to suggest that they derive more satisfaction from their sex lives than the men in Berkman and associates' study. This is, of course, a tenuous comparison, but it may suggest that in a sexual context women can more readily adapt to the loss of sensation and mobility than men. This issue needs to be studied.

Berger and Garrett (1952) believe that loss of sexual function for men is a tremendous loss and influences every aspect of life. They believe that the impact of the loss is not so much in terms of physical pleasure but in terms of a sense of inadequacy. They describe the findings in Berger's dissertation from which they conclude that impotent men with spinal injury, in comparison to sexually unimpaired men with spinal injury, were found to be more depressed, anxious, preoccupied with their own body and especially with their own genitalia, and essentially unable to enter into positive and satisfying interpersonal relationships. Teal and Athelstan (1975), in their review of the literature on the psychosocial aspects of sexuality after spinal injury, point out that Berger's study was very qualitative in nature and that Berger's conclusions were based on trends in the data consistent with his psychoanalytically oriented hypotheses.

In a similar vein and in the same era, Lindner (1953) found that impotent paraplegics gave significantly fewer sexual responses to ambiguous stimuli than persons with paraplegia who were sexually potent. He states that the impotent group showed an extreme inability to engage in vocational training or other gainful hospital occupation and showed a "narcissistic withdrawal" to preoccupation with themselves exclusively.

Both Lindner's and Berger's studies must be considered to be out of date and not really applicable to the current situation of persons with spinal injury. These gentlemen conducted their research during the early days of treating spinal injury when patients were hospitalized for years. These patients may have received the negative information customarily given in those days, and, thus, may have had good reason to be depressed. In addition, a group of men with spinal injury who retained sexual potency probably had incomplete lesions, and, therefore, their prognosis would be much less depressing than that of a person with a complete lesion.

The study by Berkman and associates (1978) tends to refute the notion that men without psychogenic erections are psychologically less adjusted and incapable of productivity and good interpersonal relationships. Thus, it is possible that able-bodied professionals could impose the requirement of mourning on persons with spinal injury in regard to sexual function. Hanson and Franklin (1976) found that rehabilitation staff viewed loss of sexual function as substantially more important to patients than patients did themselves. Consequently, Berger's and Lindner's data must be viewed with extreme caution and efforts should be made to design research to assess sexual function as one of many aspects of a person's life following spinal injury.

Whenever one considers the issue of sexual function and sexuality, the parameter of social class and cultural heritage must be considered. Kinsey, Pomeroy, and Martin (1948) found that social class was associated with differences in sexual behavior. Rainwater (1968, 1971), Bell (1969), Ferdinand (1969), and Rosenberg and Bensman (1973) describe some of the characteristics of sexual behavior among persons in lower social classes. Nudity is dealt with less comfortably, and there is great emphasis on the physical aspects of sex. Masculinity is often equated with sexual conquest, and female satisfaction is not of great concern to many of the men. Rainwater (1968) described the role of sex within lower-class families that have highly segregated sex roles versus families with less segregated sex roles. Those families that have a great separation between the roles that men play and the roles that women play were characterized by less closeness and more latent hostility between the sexes, and sex was perceived as a physical release for the man. There was little emphasis on interpersonal communication for the mutual sexual satisfaction of the couple. Families in which there was more sharing and overlap of family responsibilities showed greater closeness and more psychosocial satisfaction in sexual activity.

Certain types of sex acts may be proscribed by religious teachings, and cultural tradition may define certain activities as good and bad. In most of the studies, social class is not described but this must become a consideration in future research on sexual function.

Spinal injury may affect one's perceived desirability as a sexual partner in certain ethnic groups, and we know little about this issue. One black man with spinal injury reported that since his injury, he finds few black women who will go out with him. White women seem to find him a suitable partner more readily than black women do. Within Hispanic cultures, spinal injury may influence the range of roles a man might play within his cultural group, and this may influence his perceived attractiveness as a partner. But we do not have any data on this.

Therefore, social class and cultural heritage should be investigated as variables associated with not only sexual function but also social roles and level of participation in the community following spinal injury. And there may be sex differences within these social class and cultural heritage factors; consequently, this should be investigated.

Each one of these areas, sex drive, sex acts, and sexuality may have a primary and secondary impairment. In working with the person with spinal injury, we must evaluate the organic impairment (primary) and the behavioral implications of this impairment (secondary). Table 6.1 provides a matrix that outlines some of the parameters of sexual function following spinal injury using the conceptual frameworks proposed here. One might hypothesize that all of these issues must be considered in each individual, and the interactions among cells of the matrix are complex. This matrix may serve as a model of what should be evaluated in each person, may indicate what needs to be treated, and should be viewed as hypotheses for future research. Professionals have been dealing very globally with sexual function up to now, and our current treatment techniques seem to reflect this broad scope. However, there is a need to be more specific in our treatments and in our research in the future.

Table 6.1. Parameters of Sexual Function Following Spinal Injury

	Primary (Organic)	Secondary (Behavioral)
Sex Drive	Autonomic nervous system impairment reduces sex drive in varying degrees depending on level and completeness of lesion.	Interest in sexual activity within the context of a caring relationship.
	May find increased sensitivity of secondary erogenous zones and areas just above level of lesion.	Phantom orgasm.
Sex Acts	Loss of genital sensation and pelvic motor function.	Cultural and learned attitudes about sex acts other than genital intercourse.
	For males, reflex erections; therefore, intercourse may be difficult.	Interest in satisfying partner.
Sexuality	Physical changes in bodily appearance. Atrophy of muscles, changes in sensation, urinary appliances, use of wheelchair and orthoses, management of bowel program.	Self-image and self-esteem as a worthwhile person. Quality and nature of relationships. Repertoire of caring gestures. Ability to communicate easily. Cultural and class role expectations. Physical attractiveness.

THERAPEUTIC APPROACHES TO SEXUAL DYSFUNCTIONS IN SPINAL CORD INJURY

Hohmann (1972) has written a classic article advising professionals on how they should behave when dealing with a person with spinal injury who has a sexual dysfunction. The concepts that he presents can serve as a model of behavior for professionals no matter what therapeutic strategy is contemplated.

Beginning with the early 1970s, there have been many statements of the need for sexual counseling, but no one has presented any data as to its effectiveness in changing sexual behaviors in persons with spinal injury (Romano and Lassiter 1972; Tomko, Griffith, and Timms 1972; Romano 1973b; Miller 1975; Anderson and Cole 1975; Silver and Owens 1975; Cole 1975; Eisenberg and Rustad 1976; Evans, Halar, DeFreece, and Larsen 1976). The classic article by Romano and Lassiter (1972) describes the development of their sexual counseling program and the types of issues considered. Group sessions were held which attempted to include the partner, if possible. The emphasis was on information giving and group discussions as a vehicle to increase knowledge about the parameters of sexual functioning and to try to modify some attitudes about sexual functioning. No data were provided evaluating the effect of the program. However, this article was one of the first that described a program of this kind and that gave other professionals information regarding the specifics of a sexual counseling approach to persons with spinal cord injury.

Romano (1973b) describes the advantages of using a group procedure in sexual counseling of persons with spinal injury. Familiarity of the members or similarity to a "bull session" was one advantage, along with the opportunity for modeling. She believes that some persons find group approach less threatening, since the focus is not on themselves exclusively as it is in individual counseling. The group could serve the function of establishing norms and expectations for the members which could lead to a greater degree of participation by the members. However, she cautions that these groups were viewed as the means and context for the treatment of individuals, and use of the group to accomplish individual goals should be kept in mind.

Eisenberg and Rustad (1976) describe a sexual counseling program that consisted of eight weekly sessions, in which didactic material was presented prior to a group discussion. Two psychologists, a male and a female, conducted these groups with inputs from a neurologist. Newly injured persons were not included because it was felt that they needed three to six months to make the initial adjustment to the disability. Inpatients, outpatients, and partners were included. The content of these meetings was wide ranging, and audiovisual aids and various kinds of equipment for enhancing sexual satisfaction were presented. Individual counseling was available to all participants, if they requested it.

These counseling programs represent a positive step toward including sexual functioning as part of a rehabilitation program. Unfortunately, there is no data to assess their impact. All of the programs describe the giving of information and the sharing of experiences in groups. However, whether this leads to behavior change or "improved" functioning is not known. Are these steps sufficient to produce behavior change, or are they only the first step in a treatment program that includes multiple intervention strategies? Following these opportunities to receive the needed information about changes in sexual functioning and the desensitization group experiences can provide, the person should be seen, with his or her partner, for an evaluation of their particular sexual interaction and preferences. Then, a behavior change program should be planned and implemented, if warranted, with follow-up to determine the effectiveness of these efforts. Audiovisual aids and the book by Mooney, Cole, and Chilgren (1975) may be very helpful, depending on the particular person involved. Level of sophistication of the individual and partner, along with preinjury positive experiences with sex, would probably influence the effectiveness of therapeutic interventions in changing postinjury functioning. We need data that includes preinjury range of behaviors and postinjury range of behaviors. Measures of satisfaction from both partners regarding sex life, not about the therapy sessions, would be helpful. Romano (1973b) alludes to a reduction in the number of marital conflicts that lead to divorce or separation and an increase in satisfying social activity for unmarried participants as outcomes of group counseling regarding sexual function. Data to substantiate this observation would be very helpful in order to assist us in making treatment plans for the future.

LoPiccolo and Steger (1974) have designed and tested the reliability and validity of a paper and pencil self-report inventory for assessing the sexual adjustment and sexual satisfaction of heterosexual couples. It is called the Sexual Interaction Inventory (SII) and focuses on 17 actual sexual behaviors performed by a couple. A measure of enjoyment and satisfaction is obtained for each member of the couple across the dimension of frequency satisfaction, range of sexual behaviors, self-acceptance, pleasure obtained, knowledge of partner's preferences, and acceptance of partner. This inventory can be used as a measure of treatment outcome but has been developed using able-bodied couples. Thus, Brockway and Steger (1978) have designed and tested the Sexual Attitude and Information Questionnaire (SAIQ) for spinal injured persons and partners. The reliability has been established and the validity is currently being evaluated, using the SII as one criterion measure. Consequently, devices to assess the outcomes of sexual counseling and treatment programs are being developed and should be used by clinicians and researchers alike.

Another type of sexual program is called the sexual attitude readjustment workshop (SAR), which Cole, Chilgren, and Rosenberg (1973) adapted for use with rehabilitation professionals and persons with spinal injury. The goal is to desensationalize the participants to the various parameters of human sexuality. These workshops were introduced in order to assist health care professionals to cope with their own attitudes toward sexuality so that they would be better able to treat sexual problems in their patients. This group has played a big role in introducing sexuality into rehabilitation programs around the nation. Held, Cole, Held, Anderson, and Chilgren (1975) report the results of five such workshops. Two types of follow-up questionnaires were sent to participants. Persons with spinal injury and partners were asked if they were glad they attended the workshop (96 percent yes), if the time and expense were worth it (92 percent yes), whether the experience had been good for them personally (83 percent yes), and would they recommend it to others (91 percent yes). Professionals were sent a letter asking about their own involvement in sexual counseling (82 percent yes), and the institution's involvement in sex education for the disabled (83 percent yes). Thus, it would seem that such programs may be very helpful to professionals in rehabilitation to assist them in planning and implementing programs of sexual functioning within their rehabilitation programs.

Halstead, Halstead, Salhoot, Stock, and Sparks (1976, 1977, 1978) report similar data in using the SAR technique with combined groups of able-bodied and disabled participants. Almost all of the participants believed that it helped them personally, felt that it was worth the time and money, and recommended it for other professionals and persons with disabilities. Both groups reported that they were not as sexually active as they would like to be and cited lack of partners as the problem. The persons with disabilities were considerably less active sexually than the nondisabled group. Lack of partners was cited by 58 percent of the persons with disabilities, followed by feelings of not being sexually desirable (37 percent), and physical problems (36 percent) as reasons for infrequent sexual activity.

If health care professionals are going to be receptive to the needs of persons with spinal injury, sexual functioning must be part of a rehabilitation program. Initial data, self-report, suggest that health care professionals find SARs helpful in learning to detect their own anxieties about sexual issues, and this may make them better able to deal with sexuality in their patients. However, this remains to be demonstrated. There is no evidence that attending a SAR enhances a professional's ability to deal with sexuality. However, SAR workshops can make people more comfortable with the topic of sex. Whether this is associated with other behaviors by the professionals that help a person with spinal injury to increase his or her sexual satisfaction is not known. Perhaps SARs assist professionals in the self-selection process of whether they themselves will get involved in sexual counseling. Thus, much research must be done to assess the specific outcomes of SARs on the behavior of the professional and the disabled person. Preworkshop levels of behavior must be determined with follow-up at six-month intervals over several years. With such data, our programs can be modified to meet the needs of the participants in terms of specific behavioral goals.

The SAR technique is relatively new and its use has increased the visibility of the issue of sexual function following onset of a disability. It may be useful as a method through which professionals can become aware of their own feelings and also aware of the paternalistic attitude that they communicate to their patients. Cole, Chilgren, and Rosenberg (1973) state:

> Many spinal cord injured persons complained about the protective, fatherly attitude typically adopted by the attending physician. While this may sustain the physician's ego, it does nothing to help the patient develop his or her new self image with an altered, but functioning sense of self-sufficiency. (Cole, Chilgren, and Rosenberg 1973, p. 117)

A scale to assess attitudes toward sexuality has been developed, called the Minnesota Sexual Attitude Scale (MSAS) (Held et al. 1975; Halstead et al. 1976), and it has been used to assess changes in attitudes as a result of the SAR workshops. Such scales may be helpful in assisting us to assess the benefits of SARs, but only if combined with behavioral change data. These scales measure verbal behavior in response to the scale items, but whether actual behavior in interaction with a person in a therapeutic situation occurs, remains to be determined. Cole and Stevens (1975) assert that attitude change often precedes behavioral change. However, there is a large amount of data to demonstrate that the reverse is true (Bandura 1969). If a person changes his behavior, the cognitive and emotional responses will gradually change over time to be consistent with the new behavior. Therefore, it may be much more productive to develop behavior change strategies and then test to determine if the attitudes change over time.

If we look at SARs and counseling programs, they emphasize the giving of information and attitude change. However, whether this is the most effective method of producing behavior change remains to be demonstrated. Recently, Steger and Brockway (1978) developed a behavioral group treatment program for couples in which one member has a spinal injury. The emphasis is on behavior change in addition to the giving of information. Currently, data is being gathered to evaluate the effectiveness of the program but the initial results look promising. Hohmann (1972) alludes to an instance in which a surrogate was used to help a person overcome his anxiety regarding sexual encounters. Griffith and Trieschmann (1977, 1978) describe the use of a private room to help persons with disabilities learn to be sexual persons again while still hospitalized. They found that once the staff went beyond the discussion of the importance of sexual functioning and began to teach people how to cope with the changes in their bodies, a multibed hospital room was not an appropriate location for such activities because of lack of privacy. Thus, they used one room where a person could have privacy and be alone with another person. Including the partner in the private room experience was very helpful, since the couple had an opportunity to learn that the multiple parameters of sexuality were not affected by the onset of spinal cord injury. Some variations in sex acts might be required, but these accommodations were faced early in the disability and within the context of a complete rehabilitation program in which the partner was definitely included.

The focus in the literature is on the sexual function of the person with spinal injury, and we note the importance of including the partner in any treatment program. But there is not one study in the literature that attempts to document the reactions of the partner to the disability and to the resultant sexual dysfunction. Do partners react differently to paraplegia versus quadriplegia? Hohmann (1972) comments that many women who are responsible for the total care of their husbands with quadriplegia, including bowel care, have difficulty viewing their husbands as sexual partners. Husbands of women with quadriplegia may feel the same, if they do not have help of an attendant. It is interesting to note that Berkman and associates (1978) report that 75 percent of the men in their study said that their partners were satisfied with their sex life. It would be interesting to ask the partners.

Hohmann (1972) cautions that we should not expect too much of partners in terms of their ability to change roles. But there are no data on role changes in marriages following spinal injury and whether this is associated with sexual functioning. Much research needs to be done to identify the parameters that are important so that intervention strategies can be planned to assist couples to adjust to the disability together.

Recently, there has been increasing concern about the implantation of penile prostheses in males with spinal injury. Hohmann (1977) points out that these procedures are often performed at the discretion of the physician with little or no presurgical evaluation of the person's psychosocial status. It is not known if these devices are helpful, and, if so, to what category of persons. The data reported above indicate that many couples find sexual satisfaction without intercourse. Would a penile prosthesis enhance the satisfaction of the couple? It is not known. However, if such a device is implanted without the proper presurgical assessment of candidates and postsurgical counseling on its use, the person may never get involved with a partner to try it out. Having an erect penis does not make a ''man'' and does not ensure interpersonal satisfaction. However, this may be the implicit assumption behind a strictly surgical approach to the problem as seems to be the case in some spinal injury centers. Hohmann (1978a) is concerned that an additional assumption implicit in penile implants without proper evaluation and counseling is that it is not all right to be disabled, that rehabilitation efforts must be directed toward the transformation of the person into a pale image of the so-called normal person, the able-bodied person.

The implantation of penile prostheses without careful evaluation and follow-up of the person represents a paternalistic attitude and cannot be condoned. Therefore, it is recommended that a careful research project be designed to assess the value of such devices according to patient variables and treatment variables. Which patients find such devices helpful and under what circumstances? How do partners react to such devices? Which evaluation and follow-up procedures are most helpful to the person involved?

SUMMARY

Sexual function is a natural part of everyone's life, including the lives of people with disabilities. An evaluation and treatment program of sexual dysfunction should be included in all rehabilitation programs. Such evaluations and treatments may be facilitated if sexual function is considered to include both an organic and a behavioral component. Each of these components must be evaluated and treated in each person. In addition, it is hypothesized that all sexual function depends upon an integration of three factors, the sex drive, sex acts, and the person's sexuality. It is suggested that our efforts to assist persons with disabilities to cope with their sex lives will be enhanced if we evaluate each of these three factors.

There is some evidence to suggest that the sex drive may be diminished somewhat following spinal injury, depending upon the level and completeness of the lesion and upon the age of the person. In addition, there is some evidence that a significant proportion of marriages among persons with spinal injury succeed even though sexual intercourse may not be a frequent part of the relationship. However, there is no evidence that persons with spinal injury who do not participate in sexual relations are any less adjusted than those who do.

Our treatment efforts have been aimed at persons with spinal injury and at rehabilitation staff. Counseling, group counseling, and didactic information-giving sessions have been mentioned in the literature as methods of enhancing sexual function of persons with spinal injury and their partners. But there is no evidence to substantiate this claim. Sexual attitude readjustment (SAR) workshops have been used to help rehabilitation staff become less anxious about their own sexuality and aware of their own attitudes about sex. However, there is no evidence that the SAR approach leads to changes in the behavior of professionals in their interactions with their patients.

Therefore, we need research specifying the behavioral goal of both the counseling and the SAR approach and assessing the outcome. It is suggested that counseling and SARs may be only one approach among many, and other approaches to treatment of sexual dysfunction should be developed. Counseling and SARs may accomplish the behavioral goal of increasing the receptivity of persons to further treatment efforts and of providing the basic knowledge about human sexuality and spinal injury which is necessary for future progress. However, the assumption that counseling and SARs are the best approach to matters of human sexuality has not been substantiated. At the same time, it must be remembered that sexual function is a new area within most rehabilitation programs and within the curricula of the professions. SARs have served to increase the visibility and emphasize the importance of sexual function in the disabled person's life. Now it is time to develop the next step, behavioral techniques to teach disabled persons and their partners modes of interaction that are best suited to their conjoint interests and preinjury experiences. Research is needed to document the effectiveness of the behavioral strategies used to treat sexual dysfunctions. We need to explore the sequential or simultaneous timing of counseling and behavioral interventions. We need to explore the social class, religious, and cultural variables that influence sexual functioning. We need to examine the effectiveness of penile prostheses as a remedy of a sexual dysfunction. And we need to determine what qualifications of the staff are necessary to accomplish the various tasks involved in enhancing sexual function. There has been considerable emphasis on changing the attitudes of people in regard to sexuality. However, it is recommended that we develop strategies to change behavior and then determine, months or a year later, the effect of behavior change on attitude.

7
The Effect of the Treatment Environment on Adjustment to Spinal Cord Injury

One of the theses of this book is that rehabilitation is the process of learning to live with one's disability in one's own environment. This process of learning begins at the moment of injury and continues for the remainder of the person's life. However, the initial stages of this learning process occur within a hospital, a medical rehabilitation center, which is a complex environment composed of many behavior settings, many different personnel, and certain operational policies.

Barker (1968) has asserted that any study of behavior must attempt to differentiate between the amount of variance that reflects differences among people and the amount of variance associated with differences in environments. He asks such questions as: How do environments shape the people who inhabit them? What are the structural and dynamic properties of environments to which people must adapt? These are the questions of ecological psychology, and they have formed the basis for the work of Moos (1974, 1976) who has made an extensive study of the effects of treatment environments on patients' behaviors. Within the context of rehabilitation, and spinal cord injury in particular, Willems (1975, 1976a, 1976b) and associates have studied the patient-treatment environment interaction and have opened new avenues of research that appear to be critical to the understanding of the rehabilitation process.

Willems (1976a) believes that for a proper understanding of the behavior of the person with spinal injury, we must be aware of several principles:

1. Human behavior must be studied at levels of complexity not customary in past research.
2. This complexity relates to the *systems* of relationships of the person, the behavior, the social environment, and physical environment.

3. Such systems cannot be considered separately.
4. Such behavior-environment systems have important features that change, evolve, and become clear only over long periods of time.

Thus, in this chapter we will examine the data describing the impact of the treatment environment on patient behavior. Much of the research on the topic of spinal injury has focused on the amount of variance associated with differences among *persons* with spinal injury. Chapter 3 on the psychological variables and chapter 5 on vocational-productivity factors provide evidence of such a focus. The emphasis has been on the assets and liabilities that a person brings with him or her to the disability situation. But this is a very narrow focus, and it has been the traditional one. To better understand the process of adjustment to spinal cord injury, the effects of environments on the person with a disability must be examined. Chapter 4 on social variables attempted to outline some parameters of the social-interpersonal environment as they affect the behavior of the person with spinal cord injury. This chapter will focus on the treatment environment—the hospital, the rehabilitation center—to determine what effect it has on the behavior of the person with spinal injury.

EVIDENCE REGARDING TREATMENT ENVIRONMENTS

Miller and Keith (1973) conducted a behavioral mapping survey of patients in a rehabilitation center. The location of a patient within the hospital was noted, and the patient's activity was divided into three mutually exclusive categories: solitary, social, and treatment. Observations were made hourly over a two-week period, including weekends. The purpose of the study was to obtain an hour-by-hour record of where patients were in the hospital and what they were doing on a typical workday and a typical weekend. They found that at any one time between 8 A.M. and 5 P.M. on weekdays, exclusive of mealtimes, an average of 26 percent of the patients were in treatment areas and 60 percent were on the wards. After 6 P.M., 91 percent of the patients were on the wards. On weekends also, 91 percent of the patients were on the wards.

In terms of patient activity, between 8 A.M. and 5 P.M. on weekdays, exclusive of mealtimes, an average of 39 percent of the patients were in a solitary condition, 35 percent were engaged socially, and 26 percent were in treatment. After 6 P.M., 55 percent were solitary and 45 percent were socially active. On weekends, 66 percent of the patients were solitary, 26 percent were engaged in social interaction, and 7 percent were in treatment.

On weekends, most of the patients were in the wards and very few used the dining room or common area for socializing. They noted that Sundays in particular were times of considerable solitude with a high percentage of the patients by themselves throughout the day.

French, McDowell, and Keith (1972) describe the observations of French when he was admitted to a rehabilitation center, disguised as a patient with an orthopedic disability. He was struck by the boredom inherent in the institu-

tional routine and he noted that small events became magnified. He found that
the life of the patient was one of supervised and entirely predictable routine
with large blocks of idle time.

These data about idle time and solitary behavior of patients in a rehabilitation center document some of the concerns of Weissman and Kutner (1967)
who discuss the effects of extended hospitalization on social behavior. Because of the fixed hospital routine, the person cannot influence his environment, and he may find himself in a dependent subordinate position in regard to
the staff. In addition, hospitalization isolates a person from his family, and
patient-patient relationships are temporary and tenuous.

Further data on the interaction of the person with spinal injury and the
treatment environment has been presented by Willems and Vineberg (1969),
Vineberg and Willems (1971), and Willems (1972). Twelve persons with
spinal injury were observed continuously for 18 hours in a treatment day.
Everything that the patients did, with whom, and where was recorded for a
total of 216 hours of patient time. They found that 69 percent of the patient's
time was spent on the ward. Ninety percent of the patient time was spent in just
4 percent of the hospital's 122 behavior settings (ward, physical therapy,
hallways, and occupational therapy). Conversing, idleness, and nursing care
and hygiene represented 65 percent of the behavioral events and 51 percent of
the behavioral time in a patient day. Interactions with aides and orderlies
accounted for 41 percent of the total, followed by interactions with other
patients (16 percent), nurses and physical therapists (10 percent).

Patients' behaviors in the various settings were coded according to independence, that is, whether the patient instigated the behavior. By location, they
found that patient independence was greatest in the cafeteria and hallways and
least in occupational therapy, physical therapy, and recreational therapy.
According to type of behavior, independence was maximal in passive recreational activity (62 percent), followed by eating scheduled meals (52 percent),
transporting (48 percent), active recreational activity (40 percent), transfer-
ring (21 percent), nursing care and hygiene (15 percent), and exercise and
performance training (6 percent). Thus, they note that the highest rate of
patient independence occurred in those activities that are only accompani-
ments of comprehensive rehabilitation (passive recreation, eating, transporting), while those activities that lie at the heart of comprehensive rehabilitation
(exercise, functional training, nursing care and hygiene) produced the lowest
rates of independence.

The patients' behavior was also rated for zest, defined as instigation of the
activity and active involvement in the activity. Zest was greatest in the
cafeteria and hallways, and lowest in physical therapy and on the wards.
Categories of patient behavior and the incidence of zest were eating (68
percent), active recreational (63 percent), conversing (56 percent), transporting (50 percent), transferring (39 percent), exercise and performance training
(31 percent), passive recreational (24 percent), nursing care and hygiene (22
percent). Groups of persons involved with the patient during zestful activity

were other patients (60 percent), occupational therapists (51 percent), nurses (33 percent), physical therapists (32 percent), physicians (29 percent), and aides and orderlies (28 percent). Thus,

> The wards and physical therapy as settings, nursing care and hygiene and exercise and performance training as types of behavior, and aides and orderlies and physicians, all of which are at the heart of the formal rehabilitation process, produced the lowest zest rates. Perhaps, it is of particular interest to note that *even though zest or motivation is often seen primarily as a characteristic of persons or personalities, behavior settings, or hospital locations, do account for more of its variance than do differences among patients.* Taken together the findings on rates of patient independence and rates of behavioral zest indicate that the closer a location or activity comes to a professionally oriented definition of formal comprehensive rehabilitation, the more we initiate the activities and do them for the patient or with the patient and the more dependent, docile, and passive the patient becomes. (italics added) (Willems 1972, pp. 121-22)

Mikulic (1971) reports data on staff behavior in regard to patients that provide a clearer picture of the impact of the environment in a treatment setting. She observed the patient-staff interactions for eight patients for whom the documented goal was increased independence in self-care behaviors. She recorded the incidence of independence and dependence behaviors on the part of the patients, and the staff reaction to the behavior. For independence behaviors, the staff responded positively only 25 percent of the time and withheld positive reinforcement 72 percent of the time. For dependence behaviors, the staff responded positively 88 percent of the time and withheld reinforcement only 12 percent of the time. She concluded that the nursing personnel provided positive reinforcement more consistently for dependent patient behaviors than for independent behaviors.

Returning to the study by Albrecht and Higgins (1977) in which they measured the relationship between the various criteria of success, they note that success in rehabilitation may require that the traditional sick role, which is an institution-maintaining device, be discarded.

> After extensive observation of staff conferences, it became apparent that the medical-rehabilitation staff do not seem prepared to accept these new patient roles and therefore judge some of these independent patients to be uncooperative and not to have completed the staff's conception of the rehabilitation program. (Albrecht and Higgins 1977, p. 44)

Antler and associates (1969) report that rehabilitation staff rated the concept of wheelchair more negatively than the entire patient sample. They believe that these rehabilitation staff were reflecting a negative stereotype of the disabled by the nondisabled and that use of a wheelchair meant a loss of function rather than a positive adaptation to circumstances. One wonders if the staff's negative reaction to the wheelchair was not subtly communicated to the patients.

Taylor (1974), in a study described in chapter 3, found considerable discrepancy between the goals that occupational therapists set for persons with quadriplegia and the goals these persons had for themselves. She concludes:

> Therapists may not be communicating with patients what they perceive the goals of treatment to be or they may not be acting upon the feedback from patients regarding their wants

and goals. If it is assumed that active patient involvement in treatment is desirable, effective communication between therapists and patients is vital. Effective communication would benefit the patient in having therapy he can understand and in which he can participate to achieve mutually established goals. The patient who understands his treatment can constructively criticize it and help to describe the worth of therapy to the outside community. (Taylor 1974, p. 29)

One of the major assertions in the rehabilitation literature is the importance of having the patient as a key member of the rehabilitation team. Leviton (1973) describes the importance of the client being the comanager of the rehabilitation plan. However, Schontz (1967) reports data describing the patient conference in one rehabilitation center based on observations taken over a five-month period. The conferences involved a director, associate director, representatives of seven professional disciplines, and the client himself. Discussion of the client always began before the client entered the room and generally lasted about nine minutes. After reports were presented and a treatment plan formulated, the client was admitted to the meeting. On the average, seven minutes were spent with the patient. During this discussion the director spoke about 75 percent of the time and the client spoke about 20 percent of the time. In general, the client's comments consisted of statements of agreement with the director's proposals and instructions. The meeting was one in which instructions were given and accepted, not one in which a plan was developed through mutual exchange between client and staff.

These meetings cannot be said to encourage client co-management or independence. Indeed, this setting seems designed to coerce from clients exactly the kind of dependent unmotivated behavior that is usually regarded as prognostically poor for rehabilitation. (Schontz 1967, p. 39)

French, McDowell, and Keith (1972) report that the reaction of their participant observer to the team conference was one of feeling intimidated by the proceedings.

The number of staff involved and their proficiency at using medical terms made him feel ill at ease; the opportunity to add his opinion did not seem to be a real one since he did not feel free to talk in front of so many people. (French et al. 1972, p. 93)

These data are presented, not in order to criticize rehabilitation personnel, since they sincerely do believe that they are operating in the best interests of the patients, but in order to expand our focus as to the complexity of the rehabilitation process. Traditionally, we have focused on the person with spinal injury as the only source of motivation and as the single most important element in rehabilitation success. However, these data demonstrate that this view is too simplistic and that advances in rehabilitation will require attention to behavior-environment units.

These data suggest that rehabilitation therapies are delivered in formal, time-limited units in which the person is, indeed, the passive recipient of instructions and guidelines from the professional staff. Formal therapies permit little behavioral independence or zest, and the number of behavioral alternatives available to the patient are limited. Rehabilitation services are delivered through aides and orderlies primarily, and these are the individuals who have the least training in behavioral interaction skills. In order to accomplish their assigned duties (for example, get Mrs. M. ready for physical therapy), they often must reward dependent behaviors on the part of the patient. When not in formal therapies, much of the person's behavioral time is idle and often solitary, and, thus, Keith (1972) describes most of a day in a rehabilitation center as holding time, despite our statements about intensive treatment.

Hospitals and rehabilitation centers have been designed for the maximum efficiency of the staff, and this usually means that there are few behavior settings available to the person other than the ward and the treatment areas. Rehabilitation centers that have dining rooms for the patient are the exception rather than the rule; thus, the person eats his meal in bed. Yet we say that we are trying to train him to cope with a nonhospital world.

The data accumulated by Willems and associates demonstrates that an understanding of the patient's behavior requires an assessment of the patient-environment interaction. Lacerda (1970) has found that behavioral independence varies dramatically when patients move from one hospital setting to another. In fact, he finds that differences between behavior settings account for more variance in patient performance than do differences between patients or other variables. Willems and his group have found that a person performs differently in different settings and in addition, a person changes in different ways and at different rates, in different settings. Thus, it becomes apparent that we can no longer assess *a person's* performance. Rather, he states, we will have to assess *performance-by-settings* simply because variations in settings produce variations in performance.

Concern about the impact of the hospital environment on patient behavior has been discussed for years (Keith 1968, 1969, 1971; Kutner 1969, 1971a, 1971b; Margolin 1971; Trieschmann 1975, 1976). Margolin (1971) challenges the traditional assumption that rehabilitation failure is a result of the patient's lack of motivation. Rather, he believes that the family system, hospital system, employment system, and school system serve as deterring or facilitating factors in the person's attempts to cope with the problems of living.

Kutner (1969) describes the concept of "anti-therapy" as treatment that produces nontherapeutic results, contrary to intent. It is a phenomenon of unexpected consequences resulting in effects that are unintentionally harmful to the patient's long-term interests. Variations in patient performance from one hospital setting to another are usually attributed to insufficient training or lack of motivation rather than to variations in the behavior settings themselves.

He believes that a hospital bureaucracy is regulatory of the behavior of personnel and patients. In effect, a hospital environment is essentially a deprivational one, since the patient does not have the opportunity to perform the majority of socially determined acts whose skillful performance is at the heart of normal daily transactions. The hospital environment tends to simplify the task of being a patient. Although the patient is taught how to get well by muscle strengthening and habit training, this education occurs in a social vacuum, isolated from the demands of everyday life. In addition, he believes that professional intimidation of the patient is a subtle but fairly consistent fact of life in all hospitals. There is a tremendous social and emotional distance between patient and staff that often precludes any real participation of the patient in his own program.

Many persons with spinal injury have expressed intense frustration at the double message given by rehabilitation professionals: you must learn to be independent as a disabled person, but we will make all your decisions for you. These persons with spinal injury have described their inability to get complete information about the disability at some point, about the program planned, diagnostic or treatment procedures, medications, etc. They were expected to accept responsibility for the maintenance of their physical condition, yet they could not participate in the decision-making process regarding their own bodies (Consumer Conference 1977). Some rehabilitation personnel believe that such complaints emanate from persons who are displacing their hostility about their disability onto the rehabilitation system. Not so. These persons *have* accepted responsibility for their own lives, and they resent any efforts to interfere with their right to be informed and to participate in the decisions affecting their lives. Some of these subtly demeaning attitudes by professionals toward disabled persons have been discussed by Kerr (1970) who is one of the professional helpers and is herself disabled.

How can we best change some of these staff behaviors? Perhaps it should be part of the inservice training program at rehabilitation centers that each staff person spend two days in the role of the patient. One day could be spent on a stryker frame and the next day in a wheelchair in order to experience a typical day in a patient's life. The two-day treatment schedule should be specified for each hour of the 48-hour experience so that a standardized experience can be implemented. This would prevent the pulling of rank or special treatment that professionals might receive in the hospital. The purpose would be to sensitize professionals to the impact of their own behavior on their patients. Plans should be made to assess the professionals' behavior on multiple dimensions of patient care prior to this experience and at monthly intervals over a six-month period to determine if this experience leads to changes in their behavior. Does a less paternalistic approach to patients lead to increases in the behavioral repertoire of patients earlier during the hospital course and to more effective functioning following discharge?

AN INTEGRATION OF SOME CONCEPTS

In chapter 3, the concepts of learned helplessness and locus of control were discussed. Learned helplessness is the belief that one's behavior does not control the rewards of the environment. Locus of control is the degree of belief that one's own behavior does control the rewards of the world. It is a continuum, with externals believing in chance and fate, and internals believing in their own ability to control the rewards one gets. From the evidence presented here, it is apparent that the hospital environment is a very restrictive one in which the physical design itself limits the behavioral options available to a person, and the operational policy further limits these behavioral options. Yet, within such a system we say that we will teach a person to become independent. There is grave question as to how long we can continue to believe that this is true when we examine the data.

The early stages after spinal injury may indeed be a situation in which learned helplessness could develop. It is a highly unpleasant period and the person, in fact, has no control of what happens to him. Very gradually some degree of control is returned to the person, but it is a very limited amount of control because of the limitations of the treatment environment. Some individuals, if they are externals, may not perceive any changes in their degree of control over their environment since they expect to have very little. However, internals, those who have learned to expect control, perceive these changes and often demand more control.

Within this context, the mildly external person is viewed as the good patient because he is cooperative and does not challenge the system. The very external person gradually appears to be a problem to the staff, and he is labeled as unmotivated. He will do nothing unless it is specifically structured for him. The very internal person is perceived as a problem since he challenges the system by acting too independently and trying to make his own decisions.

We have traditionally focused on the differences among individuals, and we try to design a rehabilitation program that is uniquely suited to meet individual needs. But the individualization is in *content* of the program only. There is little individualization in *treatment approach,* depending on the person's locus of control. For example, the external person may perform best with an approach that is highly structured. Since he may not anticipate the future or work for long-term goals, the specific behavior should be specified, and rewards should be given for carrying out the assigned behavioral tasks. On the other hand, a highly structured approach may be quite ineffective for the internal person. He may perform better if allowed to set his own goals and allowed to chart his behavior to assess his progress. Up to now our treatment environment has been quite inflexible. The same approach is assumed to work for everyone. We need a much greater flexibility in our approach which essentially means making some changes in our treatment environment.

An alternative approach is to redesign the treatment environment along the lines suggested by Keith (1969, 1971). The rehabilitation process would occur in two stages, the traditional medical approach during the acute management stage and a more homelike environment in which to learn to live with the disability. Levels of assistance would be geared to the person's functional capacity. With progress, he would be expected to assume more responsibility for his own care and for the operation of the unit. He would help plan his own program and make decisions about his body and his future. The entire system would be one in which he was expected to take control of his own life, and the environment would be one that facilitated, supported, and guided such efforts.

This model, the pacemaker model, has a great deal of merit and deserves to be tested. It may be viewed with great suspicion by many professionals since it will appear to challenge their authority and competence. However, in such cases we must ask what our goals are: to provide an atmosphere that leads to best patient performance or to protect the roles that the individual disciplines have carved for themselves. We must be willing to look at our own behavior by performing research into the rehabilitation process and alternative strategies for treatment and we must be willing to consider changes in our behavior that will enhance the function of the person with spinal injury.

It is recommended that research be designed to assess the impact of various treatment environments on patient behaviors. Variations in treatment environments should be studied to determine what changes will facilitate patient performance. Variations in physical design and operational policy should be tested. Staff behavior should be examined, as part of the environment, to evaluate which behavioral approaches lead to improved patient performance. Patient variables in interaction with environment variables should be studied; to assess one without the other will be less effective in the long run.

SUMMARY

In this chapter, data are presented that suggest the treatment environment is an important variable influencing patient performance. It is too simplistic a view to attempt to assess a person's performance. Rather, the performance will be highly influenced by the environment in which it occurs.

Our goal is to facilitate patient independence through a rehabilitation program. However, there is evidence that the core features of the rehabilitation program do not, in fact, permit independence. We assess motivation by examining the patient, but the environment permits very little decision making or self-planning.

Basically, the hospital environment is designed to dispense units of treatment in an efficient manner. But dispensing units of treatment may not be the most effective approach for teaching a person to live with a disability. Furthermore, the physical design of a hospital may be inappropriate as a setting for learning to live independently. Thus, we must consider alternative approaches to the rehabilitation process, alternative models, and we must examine our current procedures and their effects on the patient.

This requires research in which professionals are willing to look at their own behavior, willing to try different ways of behaving toward patients, and willing to allow the patient to participate as an *equal* member of the team.

8
Therapeutic Techniques

Rehabilitation is the process of teaching the disabled person to live as full a life as possible within his own environment. Willems (1976a) describes rehabilitation as comprising programmatic arrangements designed to restore or substitute for lost or altered function in a person's repertoire, to teach him new forms of performance and new kinds of relations to the environment. Thus, the outcome of all of our rehabilitation efforts must be measured in behavioral terms, that is, the person's performance in naturally occurring situations over a period of time. The emphasis must be on what the person *does do* and not on what he *can do*.

> Independence is a behavioral issue because it points to performances that the person can carry out in his usual environment with a minimum of intervention and support from others. In these terms, rehabilitation means intensive and goal-oriented addition, rearrangement, and substitution in the client's repertoire of behavior and behavior-environment relations (Willems 1976a, p. 215)

Thus, the focus of this chapter will be on therapeutic techniques that lead to behavior change. Most of what occurs in rehabilitation relates to such change. The elimination of a bladder infection or bladder stone, the surgical management of a decubitus ulcer, and the traction and immobilization applied to fractured vertebrae are purely mechanical procedures designed to repair an organic impairment. But the *prevention* of bladder infections and stones, the *prevention* of decubitus ulcers and contracted joints, the *performance* of ADL and mobility techniques in order to be independent, the *practice* of social skills in relating to an attendant, family member, prospective employer, sexual partner, and clerk in the store, and the *application* of vocational skills needed to obtain and retain employment involve a multitude of individual behaviors that must be learned and practiced in order to achieve the goal of independence. These facets of independence require the learning of new behaviors, or if some of these behaviors are in the person's repertoire prior to injury these behaviors must be practiced and adapted to the new circumstances imposed by the injury. Furthermore, successful rehabilitation may require the unlearning of some behaviors that are incompatible with successful living as a person with a spinal cord injury.

The position taken in this chapter is that all psychosocial therapeutic techniques have as their goal the behavior change of the person in treatment. What behaviors are expected to change will vary and what therapeutic techniques are used to accomplish the behavior change will vary, but the ultimate goal is behavior change. The behavior changes involved may relate to insight or understanding (covert statements to oneself about one's own behavior), self-esteem or self-concept (how one presents oneself to others through verbal and motor actions and what one says about oneself), information about the disability (score on a knowledge test), prevention of medical complications, performance of ADL and mobility technique, and use of social skills in dealing with strangers. The ultimate goal of all rehabilitation efforts is also behavior change (it does no good to prescribe a tenodesus splint for a person with quadriplegia unless he finds it useful in performing some tasks he wants to accomplish). Therefore, *psychosocial therapeutic techniques are relevant to all aspects of rehabilitation and to all rehabilitation personnel*, no matter what their professional discipline.

COUNSELING AND PSYCHOTHERAPEUTIC STRATEGIES

Group counseling is a technique often recommended as a strategy to assist disabled persons in adjusting to their disabilities. Some professionals, because of their lack of specificity as to the outcomes of group therapy, seem to perceive this technique as a panacea for all psychosocial problems in rehabilitation. In contrast to this approach is the discussion of group strategies by Salhoot (1977), who presents a well-organized discussion of the application of group techniques to persons who have spinal cord injury.

Salhoot believes that group techniques have several advantages. In addition to providing a rich experience for the participants, the rehabilitation staff can gain several benefits. She believes that the group technique sensitizes the leaders to the feelings, problems, and potential of persons with disabilities in a shorter time than through individual counseling. In addition, the group experience reveals parameters of the person's psychosocial functioning that may not be apparent in individual counseling, and the feedback from group participants about the rehabilitation program assists the staff in evaluating and changing the program.

She believes that the most critical task of the group leader is to establish a specific and reasonable purpose for the group based on the needs of the participants. Many groups are unproductive because the leader and the group members are unclear about the purpose of the sessions, or the goals are so vague or broad that each person understands them differently. Thus, she describes three kinds of group strategies.

One strategy is group education which aims at developing a better basis for making judgments and decisions by examining various aspects of critical issues. In addition, this strategy can provide extensive information that the person needs to function as a disabled person. Inclusion of family members is very helpful so that they may become familiar with all aspects of the disability. The emphasis seems to be on generalized problem solving regarding many aspects of the rehabilitation program and discharge to home.

A second strategy is group counseling which is similar to the above except that the focus is on solving individual problems of group members through group interaction. She believes that increased self-understanding occurs through one's performance in the group but admits that the distinction between group education and group counseling may be hazy. It is important to specify which problems will be tackled by the group so that effort is focused on certain problems and not on all problems facing the disabled. Role playing may be helpful, and the emphasis in the group is reality-oriented and focused on the here and now. Within the group counseling strategy, groups may be formed to deal with predischarge issues, or ward management problems, or a special set of problems that happens to characterize a subset of persons at any one time.

A third strategy, according to Salhoot, is one in which audiovisual materials are used in order to provide information clearly, to provide a common experience to which group members can relate, to bring suppressed feelings to the surface about sensitive topics, and to enable productive discussions to begin rapidly. This methodology has been particularly helpful in dealing with the topic of sexual functioning, and sexual attitude readjustment workshops (SARs) use this approach.

Salhoot does not provide any data to document the usefulness of these techniques but does describe how they have been used at one rehabilitation center. Using the conceptual framework that she provides, it would be interesting to test the usefulness of these three strategies for different types of problems. However, in order to accomplish this we must define what specific behavioral outcomes are anticipated from each strategy and devise methods of measuring these outcomes.

There are two articles that describe group education programs using this conceptual framework. Lowry (1964) describes a group education program for families of persons with spinal injury within the VA system. The emphasis seemed to be very didactic with only occasional time for discussion by the participants. The outcomes that they hoped to achieve are not specified, and no data are given to assess the effect of this attempt to educate the families about the specifics of the disability. Rohrer, Adelman, Talbert, Gamble, and Johnson (1976) describe a series of one-day workshops for persons with spinal cord injury and their families. Didactic presentations, audiovisual aids, a panel discussion by former patients, and group discussion were the methodologies used during the one-day session. They report that the participants increased their knowledge of spinal injury and communication channels were reestablished among family members.

Maki, Winograd, and Hinkle (1976) report the use of a counseling-psychotherapy approach to persons with spinal injury. They advocate an ego supportive approach dealing with reality-oriented issues, believing that a more psychodynamic approach is not appropriate in the early months or years following spinal injury. However, they provide no data to demonstrate what effect their counseling program had on the patient's behavior. Manley (1973) believes that group counseling with disabled persons is a valuable tool in rehabilitation. The goal is to assist the person to gain better insight into coping with his disability. The person also has the chance to gain feelings of self-worth through group acceptance. Role playing may be used, and resource personnel may be introduced to give information on specific topics. No data are presented to assess the impact of the counseling sessions.

Mann, Godfrey, and Dowd (1973) describe a group counseling approach designed to assist each patient to increase the level of his self-concept, but they admit that it was difficult to determine if this goal was achieved. Their methodology combined many of the strategies described by Salhoot, but it seems to be a case of trying to do too much. Cimperman and Dunn (1974) describe group therapy procedures with persons who had spinal injuries. Attendance was voluntary and very erratic. Of 12 persons who indicated an interest in the group, attendance at the weekly meeting varied from 0 to 6, with an average of 3. The description of their methodology seems somewhat unfocused, and pregroup goal setting by the leaders was not apparent. No data are presented to assess the behavioral outcomes of these sessions, although an unspecified proportion of the patients thought that the sessions were valuable.

Bass (1969) describes the use of group counseling aimed at vocational adjustment for the purpose of assisting disabled persons with minimal work experience to assume, what she calls, "the worker personality." Problems encountered by this group included: inadequate social skills, feelings of incompetence, inability to get along with coworkers and supervisors, poor work habits and attitudes, and the inability to see oneself in the role of worker and to behave appropriately for this role. She describes the use of group counseling as an integral part of a program at a vocational adjustment center and states that the group is the key therapeutic instrument. Through the group experience, the participants could gain the following: old dependencies could be broken and replaced by new feelings of independence and responsibility; old values and modes of behavior could be reexamined, reevaluated, and changed, if desired; biased and unrealistic perceptions could be subjected to reality testing in the group; feelings of self-confidence and self-worth could be enhanced by group acceptance. Although the author cites the need to compare a program with and without group therapy in order to assess its impact on employment figures, she does not appear to have conducted such a study. Thus we have a proposal but no data.

Miller, Wolfe, and Spiegel (1975) conducted a study that attempted to assess the impact of group counseling procedures. They believed that persons with spinal injury might adjust better to the disability if they had adequate medical information about the impairment and shared their attitudes and feelings with others with spinal injury. The primary goal was to increase the patient's ability to cope with his disability. The effectiveness of group meetings was assessed by comparing group and nongroup members on the Spinal Cord Knowledge Inventory Test, created for the project. This instrument attempted to measure knowledge and attitude change on the facts of disability, self-concept, perceived family support, and opinion of hospital services.

Subjects were selected on the basis of their willingness to participate in the group therapy. Those who refused were placed in the nontherapy group (control group). The group met for an hour twice weekly for a period of one month. Some of the sessions provided didactic information. They found that those who participated in the group increased their knowledge about their disability and their self-concepts improved, whereas there was no change in pretest and posttest scores for the control group.

These authors should be commended for their attempt to demonstrate the effects of their therapeutic procedures. This is one of the only studies on group therapy techniques that provides some data to assess outcomes. The study has some serious methodological flaws, however, that make interpretation of the data difficult, but it does represent a beginning. Whether those who refuse to participate in therapy sessions can be considered to be a control group is questionable, since it certainly deviates from the principle of random sampling. There is no information on the test-retest reliability of the inventory constructed for this study, and we have no information on its relationship to the outcomes desired by the group therapy. In addition, in future studies it would be helpful, if not mandatory, if outcomes were assessed in operational and behavioral terms rather than by paper and pencil test. It has not been demonstrated that scores on tests of self-concept correlate highly with actual behavior in daily life.

Thus, there are a number of articles in the literature claiming that group therapy techniques are helpful to persons with spinal injury, but there are no data demonstrating this fact. Part of the problem may be the broad and often vague goals that are set for the therapy group and that may be impossible to accomplish in the time available. In addition, these goals may be impossible to measure because of the lack of behavioral specification of the outcome in question. There is no reason why good quality research cannot be conducted to assess the effects of group therapy. The usual principles of research design can be utilized and should be utilized to substantiate the many claims of its benefits.

An issue that must be considered in group counseling and individual counseling or psychotherapy is the purpose for which the therapy is initiated. Is it to present didactic information about the disability? Is it to assist in the problem solving regarding disability situations through the sharing of experiences? Is it to gain a sense of affiliation by realizing one is not alone with one's problems? Or is it to tackle psychological problems related to the experience of being disabled? In regard to the latter question, the review of the literature presented in this document does not provide any evidence that the onset of spinal injury leads to psychological problems per se. Rather the problems are reality ones, problems of learning to live in an environment designed for able-bodied people. If this is the case, perhaps the most effective therapy is the one that focuses on teaching a person to manage in such an environment.

The question of the effectiveness of psychotherapy has been discussed extensively in the literature and will not be considered here. Schofield (1964), Rachman (1971), and Frank (1974) express their doubts about the efficacy of standard psychotherapeutic techniques with a nondisabled population. Therefore, these same doubts apply to a population with physical disability. If the goal is increased ability to cope with the world outside of the hospital, it would be interesting to compare several therapeutic techniques: standard psychotherapy, group counseling, social skills and assertiveness training, and a transitional living experience with peer counseling. Which technique is most effective in producing change in which behavioral problem? Does a combination of the above techniques work better in some cases than one alone? Is there an ideal sequence of therapeutic techniques?

If we take the increase in self-confidence as an example of a frequently cited outcome of therapy, does talking about the problem solve it? Is it sufficient? It is the position taken here that talking therapy is not sufficient as a strategy to increase self-confidence and promote the ability to go out into the world and participate in a wide range of activities. Rather, self-confidence grows as the result of many interactions with various facets of the environment that are successful and rewarding to the individual. Reality-oriented talking therapy may help by assisting the person in anticipating many problems and various ways of approaching the problem. But talking about how to solve the problem may not be enough. Guided practice in problem solving through experience in the real world may be necessary if self-confidence is truly to improve. This is a testable hypothesis and should be the focus of research.

BEHAVIOR THERAPY

The term behavior therapy or behavior modification encompasses a large number of treatment strategies that have been found to be increasingly useful in a variety of behavior change situations. Applications of behavior therapy technologies have had increasing visibility in the health care field (Katz and Zlutnick 1975) and in rehabilitation settings (Michael 1970; Fordyce 1971; Berni and Fordyce 1973; Welch and Gist 1974; Cull and Hardy 1974; Kanfer and Goldstein 1975; Ince 1976; Fordyce 1976). Excellent behavioral analyses of the rehabilitation process have been written by Pigott (1969), Walls (1971), and Karan and Gardner (1973), and these should be consulted for an in-depth study of the behavioral principles operating in all rehabilitation settings. A very fine description of the impact of the onset of a disability to the individual in behavioral terms has been presented by Fordyce (1971) and should be considered mandatory reading by all who work with patients in rehabilitation. Several studies have discussed the role of behavioral principles in improving the efficiency of rehabilitation procedures: Trieschmann, Stolov, and Montgomery (1970); Sand, Fordyce, Trieschmann, and Fowler (1970); Fordyce, Fowler, Sand, and Trieschmann (1971); and Trieschmann (1975, 1976).

A major theme of this book is that rehabilitation is a behavior change process. If all aspects of rehabilitation involve behavior change, and if behavior changes according to certain experimentally established principles (Bandura 1969), then every member of the rehabilitation team (the physician, nurse, orderly, physical therapist, occupational therapist, social worker, recreational therapist, speech pathologist, and psychologist) is an agent of behavior change, and he/she should be aware of the principles of learning. If, indeed, the principles of learning govern what happens to a patient in a rehabilitation center every hour and every day, then it is imperative that we begin to explore ways to make these principles work for the patient and not against him (for example, chapter 7 described some of the unintentional effects produced by the environment on patient behavior). We will examine studies of the application of behavioral therapies to the behavior of persons with spinal cord injury in order to assess the relevance of these techniques to the rehabilitation process.

Trotter and Inman (1968) describe the use of positive reinforcement in physical therapy. They believe that although intrinsic and extrinsic reinforcers are being employed in rehabilitation, these reinforcements in general are poorly used. The reinforcers are noncontingent, not on the right schedule, or contingent on the wrong behaviors. Additional problems in rehabilitation occur, they argue, because many attempts to change behavior are based on telling or explaining the desired change to the person rather than based on altering the reinforcement environment. Thus, they wanted to determine if the planned use of reinforcement in physical therapy could promote more effective learning.

Twenty-four persons with spinal injury were randomly assigned to an experimental or control group. They were matched for level of injury, age, and onset of disability. Progressive resistance exercises to the biceps for persons with quadriplegia and to the triceps for persons with paraplegia were compared over a four-week period for the experimental and the control groups. The progressive resistance exercise program was explained to all subjects. The control group was allowed to perform their exercises independently, and no verbal or nonverbal reinforcement was planned. In the experimental group, increases in lifting were related verbally by the therapist to the subject and also related to appropriate rehabilitation goals. After ten repetitions, the subject was given a rest, praised by the therapist, and given encouragement. The lifting record was reviewed weekly with the subject and feedback was given about increases, goals, and accomplishments. The hypothesis, that planned positive reinforcement would result in greater gains in upper extremity strength, was substantiated by the data. Thus, the authors conclude that the undergraduate curricula of all rehabilitation disciplines should include training in the principles of learning. "If there is value in what has been done in this study, then these professionals need new tools for their trade" (Trotter and Inman 1968, p. 351).

Trombly (1966) describes the use of operant conditioning related to orthotic training for persons with quadriplegia. She believes that ordinary therapists indiscriminately surround the patients with encouragement and attention. The less the patient tries to be independent, the more attention he gets from the therapist who tries to convince him of the advantages of being independent. The patient discovers, however, that when he begins to try to become independent, the therapist's attention is withdrawn and he is left on his own. Thus, the therapist reinforces behavior in reverse to what the goals actually are. Trombly outlines the positive reinforcement and shaping techniques that were used to assist persons with quadriplegia to handle four different kinds of power-assisted hand splints. Unfortunately, her data were impressionistic and there was no control group.

Rottkamp (1976) assigned ten persons with spinal injury to one of two groups. One group received behavior modification training in body positioning; the other group received customary body positioning nursing care. Body positioning behaviors were modified through demonstration of body positions and shaping of body position moves. Attention from the nurse was the positive reinforcer. Following treatment, the behavior modification group showed significant differences in increased frequencies of daily changes of position and patient-initiated changes of position, decreased assistance needed for change of position, and decreased frequencies of intervals of prolonged skin pressure in comparison to the control group.

Sand, Fordyce, and Fowler (1973) describe the use of behavior therapy techniques to increase the fluid intake behavior of persons with spinal cord injury. A two-week baseline of fluid intake was established and two groups were formed: those with more than 2,500 cc input daily and those with less than 2,500 cc input daily. Part of each group were informed of the necessity of drinking more fluids, and the other part were reinforced verbally by the staff for daily increases in fluid intake and for achieving the goal of 3,000 cc daily. The group that was initially low in input but reinforced for drinking fluids increased its average daily input, whereas the informed group remained essentially the same. A battery of psychological tests and demographic variables were correlated with fluid intake behavior in the attempt to develop some predictors of drinking behavior. However, they found that a behavioral measure, low fluid input observed over weeks one and two of hospitalization, was the single most useful predictor of input later in hospitalization. They conclude that,

The present study would suggest that applying and evaluating improved training methods which assist the physically handicapped person in acquiring needed behaviors may be a more productive venture than attempting to predict occurrence or non-occurrence of these behaviors on the basis of patient characteristics. (Sand, Fordyce, and Fowler 1973, p. 261)

Malament, Dunn, and Davis (1975) describe the use of operant conditioning procedures to prevent pressure sores, using an avoidance conditioning approach. They used a pressure sensitive pad in the seat of the wheelchair. If pressure was not released by doing a pushup within a ten-minute period, an alarm would sound. By doing a pushup within the ten-minute period, the timer would reset and another ten-minute period would begin. They obtained baseline measures of pushup behavior on five persons with spinal injury and then initiated the treatment programs. There was a follow-up observation period to determine if pushup behavior was maintained without the alarm system in use. Unfortunately, the number of cases was very small (n=5), and two of the cases had to be eliminated. However, based on the three remaining cases, they found that the pushup behavior increased in frequency as a result of the training program. This research should be replicated with a larger number of cases in order to verify the findings, since it would be a very useful strategy to deal with a very costly problem, pressure sores.

Roberts, Dinsdale, Matthews, and Cole (1969) report the modification of poor personal hygiene in a person who had recurrent decubitus ulcers that had become life threatening. Twelve daily personal hygiene tasks were specified and a cup of coffee, the patient's favorite beverage, was the reward for each task performed. Each time he performed a task, he received a coupon for coffee, and coffee was not available for him without a coupon. After two months, the program was evaluated. Every day during the two-month period, he had performed each of his 12 tasks. He reported that initially he did not like the program, but later he did not object. He believed that the program had helped him. His improved hygienic behavior continued during several follow-up periods, even though he was not being rewarded with coffee. Rather, the natural rewards of the environment took over. With his healed pressure sores and improved hygiene, he was able to participate in a vocational workshop program that he enjoyed.

Taylor and Persons (1970) report an increase in time spent reading in a young man with quadriplegia who verbalized the goal of attending college but who did not engage in behaviors associated with successful performance in college. Social reinforcement by the staff was the reinforcer. Goldiamond (1973) provides a fascinating description of the behavior modification program that he applied to himself following his spinal injury.

Consequently, we have evidence that behavior therapy techniques have great utility in rehabilitation. Since all that transpires between patient and therapist is behavior modification anyway, we should be aware of the principles of learning in order to ensure that the proper behaviors are being learned and that the learning occurs most efficiently through the attachment of rewards to desired behaviors. It should be recalled that the Mikulic (1971) study showed that dependent behaviors were being rewarded inadvertently by ward staff on patients for whom the goal was increased independence.

Since all of our behavior has been shaped through the principles of learning, there is nothing intrinsically demeaning about using the behavior modification approach on patients with spinal injury. However, proper use of these strategies requires an intensive evaluation of the person so that an *individualized* program can be designed. Secondly, *rapport* between the patient and therapist is as helpful as with any of the other therapies. Instances in which the therapy program has appeared to be demeaning often relate to a violation of the above two principles. Furthermore, behavior modification programs are often introduced after all else has failed to change some behaviors, and the staff are frustrated and possibly irritated with the patient. In this context, the behavior modification program is often perceived as a punishment rather than the correct strategy that should have been utilized in the very beginning.

There are not too many published reports of behavior modification with persons who need to learn the behaviors necessary for survival with a spinal injury, but there is a voluminous literature on the use of these techniques with many types of behavior problems. Much of this literature may be applicable to rehabilitation in general and spinal injury in particular. The work on self-control procedures by Kanfer and Karoly (1973) and cognitive behavior modification by Meichenbaum (1977) hold great promise for rehabilitation. The work by Willems (1976b) and associates is very relevant since, in most behavior modification programs, it is a change in the environment that leads to a change in the person's behavior. Actually, almost all behavior modification programs require changes in staff behavior in order to produce changes in the patient's behavior. Perhaps this is why many professionals find behavior modification techniques so very threatening and upsetting. *It forces us to face the fact that our customary ways of behaving toward the patient do not produce the desired results.*

Changing the behavior of staff members is a customary feature of most behavior modification programs because these programs involve rearranging the environment to reward the patients and the staff constitute a critical feature of the environment. Thus, attention should also be given to means of improving the patient-staff interaction.

Sadlick and Penta (1975) found that viewing and discussion of a videotape of a person with quadriplegia who was successfully rehabilitated improved student nurses' ratings of their attitudes toward persons with quadriplegia. This effect persisted, but diminished somewhat, during the nurses' ten-week training with spinal injury in a rehabilitation ward. Although their own attitude about themselves working with persons with quadriplegia improved after the film and discussion, this effect did not remain at the end of their rotation through the rehabilitation ward. The authors believe that this may relate to the discrepancy between the level of function of the patients on the ward who were early in the initial rehabilitation phase and those seen in the film.

There are a number of studies demonstrating that the rewarding of staff for patient improvement leads to greater degrees of patient improvement than the usual situation in which staff rewards (salary, promotion, etc.) are not necessarily related to improved patient function (Pomerleau, Bobrove, and Smith 1973; Loeber 1973; Pommer and Streedbeck 1974; Sand and Berni 1974). This is, of course, a touchy issue since most persons who work in rehabilitation centers are sincerely concerned about the welfare of their patients and believe that they are doing the best that they can to facilitate patient improvement. However, these studies suggest that despite our sincere intentions, our strategies may need to be changed as suggested by Trotter and Inman (1968).

Much research is needed to determine what types of behavior therapy techniques are best for particular behavior change problems. We should also outline a comprehensive research program to determine if planned use of behavior therapy techniques leads to more efficient learning, considering the spiraling cost of rehabilitation care. We need studies with a large enough sample and a control group in order to assess the effectiveness of these approaches. We need to examine the effect of including courses on the principles of learning in the curricula of all rehabilitation professionals, along with inservice training for aides and orderlies who spend so much time with the patient. Most of all we need to specify target behaviors for all patients which can be used to define outcome or success. These behaviors need to be observable and countable. In this way, we can assess the effects of different treatment approaches and measure the quality of the rehabilitation program.

SOCIAL SKILLS TRAINING

Many individuals with spinal injury are discharged from rehabilitation centers with no training or practice in the social skills that are necessary to cope with the devaluation they will experience from able-bodied persons. Cogswell (1967, 1968) describes the process of self-socialization that persons with spinal injury experience. She found that upon discharge, and in comparison to preinjury life, all the persons with spinal injury in her study had a marked reduction in the number of social contacts with others in the community, the frequency of entering community settings, and the number of roles they played. All in her sample eventually showed some increase in social activity, but the extent of the increase was highly variable. She claims that persons with spinal injury know what their goal is, reintegration into the community, but they have no awareness of the steps needed to obtain this goal. There is no one to spell out or to structure the progress toward this goal.

Romano (1976) recognizes the need for social skills training and outlines the facets of such an approach. She advocates the use of behavioral rehearsal and assignment in which people must consider a given situation and the different kinds of response, and then must practice their chosen response with feedback. She recommends the use of shaping and successive approximations to the final goal by arranging tasks graded by difficulty, with advancement to each step contingent on accomplishment of the previous step.

Recently, Dunn (1977) devised a social discomfort scale which he used to rate the degree of discomfort a person has about a range of social situations (see chapter 4). In addition, he and his associates have created a film that depicts eight potentially sensitive social situations involving disability. Each situation is depicted with three styles of response: aggressive, passive, and assertive. Each scene is followed by a commentary identifying the important behavioral and verbal components of the different responses. The commentary emphasizes that it is up to the person in the wheelchair to help people become more comfortable with the handicap, that a person with spinal injury who acts like a "cripple" will be treated like one, and an active, assertive approach is more likely to produce a favorable outcome for all parties involved.

Dunn, Van Horn, and Herman (1977) describe a research project using this film in a social skills training program. Group 1 (six subjects) had a four-week, eight-session training course involving videotape feedback, lecture and discussion, and modeling in learning to manage the eight situations depicted in the film. Group 4 (four subjects) had the same experience as Group 1 but, in addition, saw one segment of the educational film at the end of each session that dealt with that subject area. Group 2 (six subjects) was shown the entire film on one occasion, four weeks after the start of the study. Group 3 (six subjects) received no intervention. Assessment before and after the treatment program consisted of the social discomfort scale (paper and pencil) and a videotape measure of performance.

There were no significant differences among the groups on the paper and pencil test, but on the videotape of performance, Groups 1 and 4 were significantly more assertive than Groups 2 and 3. There was some evidence to suggest that Group 2, which saw the film only with no discussion, showed an increase in anxiety. This raises the concern that training programs of this kind may need to be made more complete, to include discussion and practice, and not only to inform a person about the number of alternatives available. Studies on populations other than spinal injury indicate that instructions, feedback, and modeling in combination lead to greater increases in components of social skills than any one of these techniques alone (Edelstein and Eisler 1976; Hersen and Bellack 1976).

Thus, this work by Dunn and associates seems to be promising as one approach that can assist the person with spinal injury to overcome the social anxiety that was so apparent in Cogswell's study. This is an excellent first step; more training programs need to be developed and research conducted to document the outcome. It should be remembered, however, that our ultimate goal is not to change scores on a paper and pencil test but to change performance in actual social situations. Furthermore, the optimal length of these training programs and the timing of these programs within rehabilitation need to be determined. Are several courses spaced over time more efficient than presenting everything at once? One might predict that such social training may not lead to changes if the person has few naturally occurring social interactions available. Thus, follow-up research should differentiate between groups who have had a chance to practice their social skills and those who have not. The literature on assertiveness training and social skills training using a nondisabled population will be helpful as leads for new programs and research into this area.

Structured learning therapy is a technique described by Goldstein (1973) as a psychotherapy for the poor. He believes that middle-class clients and middle-class therapists enjoy the traditional type of therapy that emphasizes introspection, verbal exchange, search for insight, and nondirectiveness from the therapist. However, the less verbal person is going to be less enthusiastic about extensive verbalization since he has come to the therapist to be given solutions to his problems. A more authoritarian approach by the therapist is what is expected. Therefore, Goldstein believes that traditional psychotherapeutic procedures are less appropriate for this type of person, and he prefers structured learning therapy which entails modeling, role playing, and social reinforcement. The emphasis is on the here and now, and reality problems are tackled.

This type of approach may have considerable merit for persons with spinal injury since many are more action-oriented than verbally oriented, regardless of level of intelligence or social class. These components—modeling, role playing, and social reinforcement—seem to appear in various therapeutic approaches and probably will become the core of future psychosocial approaches.

Roessler, Milligan, and Ohlson (1976) describe an approach called Personal Adjustment Training (PAS), a structured group counseling approach for persons with spinal injury. The program attempts to teach participants to improve their interpersonal relationships, their ability to identify and set priorities, their ability to specify steps toward achievement of a goal, and their ability to act toward goal achievement. Although the authors attempted to conduct a research project to assess the value of PAS, using an experimental and control group, they were not able to complete the study because of the 60 percent to 80 percent attrition rate of subjects. The attrition rate was high because PAS was never considered to be an important priority in the rehabilitation program by the remainder of the staff. Subjects missed PAS sessions because other appointments were scheduled at the same time, or they were held over by previous appointments and were late to the PAS sessions. Furthermore, the completion of the physical or occupational therapy program or the vocational training program was the signal for discharge from the center despite the fact that they had not completed the PAS program. This type of a program seems to have merit conceptually and deserves the chance to be evaluated properly.

However, the experience of those authors identifies a persistent problem in rehabilitation centers. Physical rehabilitation activities take top priority whenever there is a schedule conflict. Psychosocial rehabilitation activities are considered superfluous. Therefore, we need to test this question: a group of persons with spinal injury who have the usual physical rehabilitation approach only should be compared with those who have social skills and assertiveness training, and any other psychosocial treatment strategy, in addition to the physical rehabilitation program. Ability to function in the world one year after discharge would be evaluated for these two groups. It is time to test the merit of psychosocial training following spinal injury and determine if it has any value. Merit in this case would be defined as performance of a wide range of behaviors in the world and the incidence of fewer medical complications. The hypothesis is that psychosocial rehabilitation enhances one's ability to function in the world and increases the probability that one will find some rewards and satisfactions following onset of disability. If one has some rewards and satisfactions in life, then one will be more likely to take care of one's body and prevent medical complications.

The issue of timing becomes important along with the issue of the amount that we can expect a person to learn at one time. The concept of massed practice versus spaced practice is relevant also. Is it efficient to include social skills training during the initial inpatient rehabilitation phase or do we need a two-stage approach to rehabilitation? Considering the fact that chapter 7 expressed concerns about the impact of the hospital environment on patient behavior, is such a setting the appropriate place to teach self-management, assertiveness, and the skills to cope with an extrahospital environment? Perhaps, following the physical rehabilitation, the person should graduate to stage two (not to imply secondary but more advanced), wherein he can learn to apply his new ADL and mobility skills in an atmosphere, such as a transitional living center, that encourages self-management.

MILIEU THERAPIES

Kutner (1968) describes milieu therapy as a theory of treatment and a body of associated methods in which the environmental or residential setting is utilized as a training ground for patients to exercise social and interpersonal skills and to test their ability to deal with both simple and complex problems commonly experienced in open society. The approach is particularly helpful with those patients who adapt all too readily to hospital life and assume the dependent, chronic, invalid role too easily. Such programs have the advantage of preparing the person for the demands of the extramural environment so that discharge does not lead to a decline in behaviors emitted.

Abramson, Kutner, Rosenberg, Berger, and Wiener (1963) describe such a therapeutic community in a hospital rehabilitation service. The patient should participate in the decision making regarding his program, and he should assume increasing amounts of responsibility for his own care. Hospital visiting hours can be made more flexible to include the family and friends more readily. Extended home visits and participation in out-of-hospital social events help to prevent social isolation. It is not clear if this program was implemented as described and we have no information on its success or failure.

Some of these procedures have been introduced gradually into other programs. Johnson, Roberts, and Godwin (1970) report the implementation of a self-medication program on their ward, and Becker, Abrams, and Onder (1974) report a joint patient-staff method of setting goals. None of these reports provides data that allow us to compare the new approach with the old one, however. Therefore, these remain in the realm of suggestions for future research.

Keith (1969, 1971) calls for alternative models of rehabilitation care, such as the pacemaker model. He proposes a residential unit in which patients accept as much responsibility for the management of the unit as they are capable of. Sections of the residence would be graded by the amount of assistance that is available. As patients progress in gaining degrees of function, they would graduate to the next section in which less help is available, and the patient has to accept more responsibility for the maintenance of his environment. At the highest levels of independence, cleaning, laundry, and food preparation would be part of everyday life, in addition to other ADL tasks. An essential ingredient in Keith's proposal is understaffing, based upon the finding of Barker (1968, 1976) that understaffed environments lead to more independence, more acceptance of responsibility, and to a larger number of tasks performed by each person. This concept within rehabilitation should be tested. However, the gradual evolution of transitional living centers is one step in this direction.

CHEMOTHERAPY

The use of major chemotherapeutic tranquilizing agents soon after the onset of spinal injury to assist the person to cope with the emotional aftermath of the injury can be a controversial issue. Few physicians who are skilled in the treatment procedures of spinal injury advocate such a course of action on a routine basis. However, it is an unfortunate fact that some physicians who have the responsibility for treating persons with acute spinal injuries do, indeed, prescribe major tranquilizers routinely to counteract the "massive depression" that they believe follows the injury (Romano 1978).

However, there is no evidence that the onset of spinal cord injury leads to psychotic reactions except in the extremely small percentage of cases in which there was evidence of profound behavioral disruption prior to onset of the injury. Transient states of disorganization caused by sensory deprivation remit as a result of increased sensory inputs rather than through the use of pharmacological agents. Furthermore, evidence tends to suggest that most persons with spinal injury do not suffer "massive depression," although some depression is apparent in many. What depression occurs is related to a reality event about which most people are decidedly unhappy. Therefore, the question arises: Is it necessary or appropriate to prescribe drugs to dull one's perception of the unhappiness of the event?

Most clinicians who are experienced in the treatment of spinal injury find that chemotherapeutic intervention is not necessary except in the small percentage of cases that exhibit signs of a preexisting psychosis or the classic signs of a severe depression: loss of appetite, insomnia, and psychomotor retardation. A pharmacological agent that acts as an energizer and appetite stimulant may be helpful to get the person going until some of the natural rewards of progress in rehabilitation begin to maintain the person's behavior.

At this time it is the opinion of a large number of physicians who are nationally prominent in the treatment of spinal cord injury that the routine prescription of major tranquilizers is not appropriate (Young 1978). However, research using double blind procedures would be helpful to test the question of the efficacy of chemotherapeutic agents as treatments of the emotional concomitants of spinal cord injury.

ALTERNATIVE MODELS OF SERVICE DELIVERY

In recent years there has been a growing realization that physical rehabilitation procedures carried out in a hospital setting may not prepare a person adequately for the demands of life outside of the hospital. As a result, some new approaches to rehabilitation have evolved that relate to both Kutner's (1968) and Keith's (1969, 1971a, 1971b) suggestions regarding rehabilitation environments.

Manley and Armstrong (1976) describe a transitional living facility that is part of a regional spinal cord injury center. The facility consists of a 20-unit apartment building, each unit accessible and furnished for wheelchair use. The original purpose for the facility was to provide a low-cost environment for persons with spinal injury who were returning to the center for a follow-up evaluation. A stay in the hospital for this period would cost 400 percent more than residence in this facility. This finding has great implications for the cost of follow-up care. However, in addition, the facility has been used for a two-week practice session of the skills learned in the rehabilitation program. The patient and family can live together, identify any areas of difficulty in functioning, and gain self-confidence while maintaining a close contact with the rehabilitation center. A comparison of those discharged to the apartment complex and those discharged directly to home showed that individuals and families who have had the benefit of the living experience program have fewer medical complications and seem to encounter fewer problems in reestablishing family roles.

Another project that seems promising is a cooperative living program (Stock and Cole 1977) which has evolved into the New Options Program at one of the regional spinal cord injury centers. A building that had been originally intended to serve as an extended care facility was purchased. Forty persons with paraplegia and quadriplegia entered the program during the project period. Most had been living at home with family and were unemployed, or were residing in a nursing home. The average level of monthly income at admission was $122.00. Most persons required assistance with a certain number of activities, and, thus, students were hired as attendants and the help was shared among the patients. A resident council and resident manager were in charge of the organization, and social-interactional problems among the residents were handled by the council. Each resident had a private room and was responsible for scheduling time for attendant care.

During residence at the facility, the day's activities consisted of modules that were designed to impart information and provide practice at coping with the demands of the world. Financial management and budgeting, use of public transportation, field trips to employment locations and community facilities were among the activities. Attendant management, home management, problem solving, sexuality, medical needs, leisure time use, mobility, educational and vocational opportunities were also included as modules. The residents had a wide variety of opportunities to socialize in many settings.

The results of this transitional living program are impressive. Based on 40 residents, 53 percent of the sample had an income of less than $100.00 monthly before admission. As of January 1977, only 5 percent of the participants had an income of less than $100.00 monthly. The average income prior to admission to the program was $122.59 monthly, and, as of January 1977, the average income monthly was $496.91. This change in income was related to change in employment status. Prior to entry in the program, 1 person was employed full-time and 4 part-time. The level of income of the 14 residents employed full-time reflected the shift to economic independence. Prior to the program, the average income of these 14 persons was $1,447 annually, or $129.99 monthly. As of December 1975, the average annual income of these persons was $7,560 and $630.00 monthly, an increase of 488 percent. Three of the individuals who were employed full-time after the program had been residents of nursing homes prior to the program. These data are particularly impressive because the figures in December 1975 reflect actual earnings since the individuals were no longer eligible for agency support. In addition, these data substantiate the claim of Edward Roberts (1976), director of the California State Department of Rehabilitation, who believes that it is counterproductive to get a person involved in a vocational rehabilitation program aimed at full-time employment until he or she has had a chance to master the skills necessary for survival in the community. The usual inpatient rehabilitation program does not teach the person these skills nor does it offer the opportunity to practice social and survival skills in the community prior to discharge. Thus, the rehabilitation process seems to require several years for the average person.

The data that Stock and Cole (1977) present comparing the cost of living in various environments should be helpful for future planning. They compared the monthly living costs in Houston, Texas, as of November 1975, for four types of living environments. They found that monthly expenses for a nursing home were $743.00; for an apartment with a private attendant, $840; for an apartment with shared services, $660; and for the cooperative living project, $570. On the basis of this data, it seems that cooperative living projects may be a very worthwhile investment in the client's future. In addition, for individuals without homes and little probability of vocational and financial independence, a cooperative living situation may be a more cost effective living arrangement than nursing home placement.

This was the conclusion of the Handicapped Persons Pilot Project (1969), sponsored by the California State Department of Public Health. An assessment of the survival needs of severely disabled persons was made, and the costs were compared for providing these needs within the context of an institution (hospital), an extended care facility (nursing home), or a boarding home. The latter option was much less expensive than the former two alternatives. Thus, we would recommend that boarding homes or cooperative living centers be created as an alternative for those disabled persons who cannot live independently, cannot live with family, and do not need a nursing home. However, these should not be custodial facilities, but rather community living experiences in which each resident is expected to participate in the operation and management of the center. Several cooperative living centers should be established, and the costs should be compared with nursing home placement. These cooperative living centers would serve as the residence for most of the participants, although if an opportunity for independent living appeared, the person would be encouraged to try it. However, the transitional living center, in contrast, would emphasize a limited period of residence during which the person was in training for living on his own.

Barrie (Professional Conference 1977), who for 30 years was chief claims agent for a major private insurance company, learned that he saved his company a tremendous amount of money if he financed the costs of postdischarge adaptation to life. He found that it was penny-wise and pound-foolish to finance only the inpatient rehabilitation phase and then to confine future expenditures to a pension plus hospital expenses because of medical complications after discharge. By investing money in the home and family situation so that the person could maximize his independence and not be a tremendous drain on the family, a number of medical problems and the resultant cost of rehospitalization were reduced. By helping the person find some satisfactions and rewards in life, the number of medical complications caused by neglect dropped in frequency and yearly hospitalization costs were reduced.

One feature of this program, which Barrie believes accounted for its success, was the case manager approach (Barrie 1973). One person within the insurance company was assigned to manage the person's case. This nonmedical person was responsible for overseeing the person's rehabilitation from the moment of injury and for the rest of the person's life. Medical rehabilitation and psychosocial services were selected that were designed to enhance the disabled person's functioning, and services were sought that indeed accomplished this goal. The case manager was fiscally responsible for management of the person's entire program; therefore, costs did not increase through fractionation of care and periods of neglect. Money was spent to make the disabled person's life more comfortable (purchase of a car with hand controls, electric typewriter, etc.) because this expense for psychosocial comfort was offset by lowered future hospitalization bills associated with self-neglect and medical complications.

The case manager approach has been adopted by the state of Arkansas which has created a Spinal Cord Injury Commission that reports directly to the governor. A rehabilitation counselor, with special training in spinal cord injury, is assigned to be the case manager of each newly injured person and follows this person from injury onward. The case manager has the fiscal responsibility of obtaining the services needed to enhance the functioning of the person with spinal injury (Carmack 1977). This approach should be studied, and the costs of rehabilitation using the case manager approach versus the usual approach in state departments of rehabilitation should be compared for a ten-year period. It may turn out that we can no longer afford the fractionated care and limited services that a large proportion of the spinal injury population receive (Professional Conference 1977).

The state of Alabama has initiated a Homebound Rehabilitation Program financed by the state legislature and initiated through the efforts of Governor George Wallace. Any severely disabled person is eligible for services. There are no age limitations or eligibility for employment requirements. Medical assistance is provided, when indicated, including hospitalization and treatment. Attendant care, home modification, and procurement of special equipment and supplies through purchase or loan are available. A key feature of this program is the home health team which visits persons in their homes to teach them and their families to deal more successfully with their disabilities. Better health habits are taught in addition to special exercises, skin care, and prevention of medical complications. Each home health team consists of a counselor, a registered nurse, a physical therapist, and a secretary. The team works with local physicians and has medical consultants available. Also, they work with the local agencies and hospitals. The state is divided into six regions, and there is a home health team for each region.

Both Alabama and Arkansas have initiated highly innovative programs of service delivery which need to be examined and evaluated. Thus, we should plan research to document the outcomes of new approaches to service delivery such as the case manager approach, homebound programs, transitional living centers, and cooperative living centers. These programs could complement the regional spinal injury center network.

INDEPENDENT LIVING CENTERS

In recent years, there has been an increased interest by persons with disabilities in the provision of services to other individuals with disabilities. This interest has arisen because many disabled persons believe that their experiences in rehabilitation centers have not equipped them to meet the demands of life outside of the hospital. Thus, independent living centers have developed around the United States, based somewhat on the model established by the Center for Independent Living (CIL) at Berkeley, California.

These centers are staffed by persons with disabilities and usually are non-residential in nature. Wheelchair and equipment repair services, attendant referral services, disability stipend counseling, home modification services, accessible housing surveys, transportation services, referral services, and peer counseling are among the kinds of activities that may be offered by any one center. In addition, the Berkeley CIL provides training for rehabilitation counselors on the survival needs of persons with disabilities.

Peer counseling is an interesting facet of these programs. Persons with disabilities can advise others with disabilities how to cope with various reality problems, based on their own experiences. Thus, modeling is possible since the centers are staffed with competent people with severe handicaps who have succeeded in handling the daily problems of living. Furthermore, these centers have played an advocacy role for the person with a disability; they try to determine what benefits are available to the person and how the person can obtain these benefits. It will be interesting to note whether these programs may be able to influence community attitudes by challenging the stereotype of the disabled person as needing pity and constant assistance from nondisabled people.

What effects these centers will have remains to be determined, and research should be initiated to document the outcome of their services. Clearly, they have been developed to meet some needs currently unmet. Therefore, the question arises as to whether there are some services that can be performed best by disabled persons rather than by professionals who are not disabled. Most members of these organizations believe that the answer is yes. Therefore, this should become an issue for research. Currently, there are no data to evaluate the influence of peer counseling and there are no clear guidelines as to what constitutes peer counseling or the type of training procedures best suited to train peer counselors. In addition, when does peer counseling end and more traditional psychological counseling begin? If these centers do deliver psychological counseling services by nonprofessional (and nonlicensed) persons, is this detrimental to the client? These last issues can become touchy, and the legalities of the activities (depending on state licensing) may become complex. Nevertheless, it seems that independent living centers can be a viable force in the community, and their activities should be evaluated through a well-defined program of research.

A similar concept has been proposed by Hohmann (Professional Conference 1977) who believes that a tutorial method may be very helpful with newly injured persons. He proposes that the person with spinal injury, upon discharge from the rehabilitation center, go to live for several months with a person who is experienced in living with the disability. At the end of this period, he believes, the recently injured person will be much more sophisticated in his ability to cope with the world. Modeling is inherent in this approach and in the independent living programs. Modeling would also be possible if persons with spinal injury were hired, when qualified, to fill positions at regional spinal cord injury centers or other rehabilitation centers. When the newly injured person is told that a full life is possible despite the disability, the sight of persons with spinal injury functioning within the world will add meaning to such prognostications. Thus, we should specifically research ways in which modeling can aid in the rehabilitation of persons with spinal injury.

SUMMARY

There are many articles that discuss the benefits of group therapy, but there is not one that provides any evidence to substantiate this claim. Group counseling techniques may be an efficient method for having several persons share ideas and explore new ways of coping with a disability, but we need research to test this question. Group counseling or therapy that focuses on developing insight and improving self-esteem seems to be implicitly based on the assumption that onset of disability leads to psychological problems per se; however, there is no evidence that this is true. Logically, it seems more effective to improve self-esteem and confidence by experiencing success in coping with the real world. Thus, programs to teach people the skills they need to do this should be the focus of rehabilitation.

Behavior therapy programs have been studied as methods of increasing fluid intake, changing bed position, doing pushups, increasing upper extremity strength, improving personal hygiene, and facilitating other activities related to improved function. Data show that behavior modification programs do work when carefully planned and executed. Therefore, since rehabilitation is a learning process and all that happens within the rehabilitation center is focused on modifying the behavior of the person with spinal injury, it seems obvious that the principles of learning should be used to produce this behavior change in the most efficient manner possible.

Social skills training and assertiveness training have been studied only recently and deserve to be the focus of much more research. Persons with spinal injury need to be taught ways of coping with a social world that is often rejecting and cold. Whether this training can occur most efficiently within the present hospital system needs to be studied. The two-stage approach to rehabilitation needs to be researched: physical rehabilitation within the traditional rehabilitation center, and psychosocial training in a transitional living center, for example.

Alternative models to the current rehabilitation center should be considered and studied to determine their efficiency in producing behavior change. A self-management type of center, transitional living centers, independent living centers, and tutorial models should be examined. The case manager approach and homebound rehabilitation programs should be studied as complements to the regional spinal injury centers.

Thus, the concepts in this chapter hold the key to future advances in the state of the art. Rather than trying to identify winners and losers, we should develop strategies to teach the multitude of skills needed to live with a disability and study the outcomes of these strategies.

9
Adjustment to Spinal Cord Injury: An Overview

The review of the literature and of expert opinion reveals the fact that there are tremendous gaps in our knowledge about the process of adjustment to spinal cord injury. These gaps are particularly distressing since there is data to suggest that between 12 percent and 46 percent of the deaths of persons who survive the acute phase of spinal injury may involve self-neglect or self-destructive behaviors. Most of these deaths occur within five years of injury. Therefore, since our rehabilitation efforts are not completely successful, it is important to study the process of adjustment and the process of rehabilitation in order to identify appropriate behavioral goals and effective intervention strategies to accomplish these goals.

Much of rehabilitation in the past has utilized the medical model which is essèntially a units of treatment approach. This may be successful in treating acute disorders; however, with chronic disabilities such an approach may be counterproductive because the person must be a passive recipient of the treatments dispensed. Thus, there is an inherent conflict between the medical model and the goals of rehabilitation which are to teach a person to function in his or her own environment. As a result, an alternative model of rehabilitation, the learning model, is proposed, since it is much more consistent with the goals of rehabilitation. In this approach, rehabilitation is viewed as a learning process in which the behaviors needed to cope with the nonhospital world are taught by teachers (rehabilitation staff) using the principles of learning. To use this' model effectively, behavior must be viewed as the complex result of person, organism, and environment variables. In fact, it is proposed that the key to the rehabilitation process is the arrangement of person-environment interactions that promote the behavioral goals desired. To accomplish this task, the person and environment variables influencing behavior must be identified, and intervention strategies must be developed that increase the person's ability to function in his or her own environment. Unfortunately, however, most of the literature to date has dealt with person variables exclusively.

There is little information reliably demonstrated about the immediate consequences of spinal injury. Speculation persists, however, that the early weeks, perhaps months, involve a state of psychological shock in which the person actively denies what has happened. But no data have been found to substantiate this notion. Rather, it is hypothesized that any clouding of the sensorium during the acute stage results from a combination of circumstances: anesthesia from surgery, medication for pain, sensory deprivation, and sleep disruption. Consistent with this hypothesis is the fact that a large percentage of patients actively desire information about their injury and its implications within two weeks of onset.

The literature is full of articles describing *the* stages of adjustment to spinal injury, and the same unsubstantiated ideas are repeated like a litany. The stage theory of adjustment proposes that the immediate reaction to disability is denial, followed by profound depression, which is replaced by alternating feelings of hostility and dependency. It is proposed that a person must go through these stages and mourn one's predicament in order to become adjusted to the disability. Furthermore, it is feared that the adjustment process will not be complete until the person has experienced depression and truly mourned the loss.

However, the data suggest the opposite. Recent research tends to suggest that those who are least depressed tend to function best during rehabilitation and following discharge. Those who do become significantly depressed may do much less well after discharge. There is no evidence of stages of adjustment at this time, and only mild depression during the second or third week has been noted. Thus, depression, in a classic sense, may be the wrong term to describe the reaction to spinal injury. Unhappiness may more precisely describe this state.

Research that documents the emotional reaction to spinal injury is complicated by the finding that spinal injury may reduce the experience of emotional feelings because of disruption of the autonomic nervous system. The higher the level of the lesion, some believe, the greater the reduction in experienced emotional feelings. Patients have reported, however, that they often act "as if" they were feeling emotional, because it is expected of them by those around them, and they get attention for their requests. Consequently, to study the emotional reaction to spinal injury, multiple levels of measurement must be used including a biochemical measure and several direct behavioral measures of emotion. Rehabilitation staff are not good observers of psychological processes, and ratings by staff consistently overestimate the degree of psychological distress present. Furthermore, longitudinal research seems to be the more effective way of reliably determining the fluctuating role of emotions in the adjustment process.

Motivation has been viewed as the key to the rehabilitation process. If the patient is motivated, he or she will be a success. However, motivation is looked upon as a drive within the individual to get better and is often synonymous with cooperation with rehabilitation staff decisions. Within this view, the emphasis in the literature has been on the identification of those with motivation and on the attempt to screen out those with a deficit in motivation. However, there is no remedy for a motivational deficit within this approach, and psychotherapy has proved unsuccessful.

On the other hand, if motivation is regarded as those rewards and satisfactions in the environment for which the person will work, it is external to the person and capable of being influenced by rearranging the environmental rewards. There is much evidence that this approach works, and "unmotivated" patients can change their behavior through the use of behavior therapy techniques, thus giving credibility to this view of motivation.

Locus of control seems to relate to the concept of motivation, and it may become a core concept in working with the disabled person. Persons with an external locus of control tend to become more depressed following spinal injury and to do less well after discharge. Those with an internal locus of control show less depression and function very well following discharge. Locus of control relates to the degree of belief that one's behavior controls the rewards of the world. Externals believe in fate, luck, chance, and powerful others, and may be more susceptible to the experience of learned helplessness. The onset of spinal injury may be one of the most extreme examples of helplessness in the natural environment, and if some persons are susceptible to learning that they are helpless to control the rewards of the world, they may function very poorly in the rehabilitation center and after discharge. Thus, it appears that the behavioral view of motivation and the concepts of locus of control and learned helplessness may provide a key to the improved functioning of a large percentage of persons with spinal injury.

Body image as a traditionally defined personality variable has not been demonstrated to relate to the adjustment to disability. However, body image as the sensory response to parts of one's body, has been shown to be disrupted in a large percentage of persons with spinal injury soon after onset. The perception of the body in positions other than the one visually noted is the most common experience. These body image distortions tend to disappear in a large proportion of persons within several months of injury.

Pain is a frequent experience immediately after the injury but tends to disappear within several weeks unless there is scarring from extensive surgery or unless the person is not managed well in the early stages. There is some evidence to suggest that persons who have not received proper psychological management may have more pain complaints than those who have received proper care. The correlation between the incidence of pain complaints and a prior history of alcohol or drug abuse is suspected but not proven.

Demographic variables may be quite influential on function following spinal injury. There is some evidence that the young person adjusts somewhat better than the older person, and the age range 20–35 may have the greatest variability in ultimate functioning. There is no evidence that severity of disability per se influences adjustment. Rather, person and environment characteristics play a more important role in determining outcome. We have no evidence on the influence of duration of disability, although it appears that it may take two to four years to learn to live with the disability with some degree of comfort and satisfaction. Sex may be a variable in ultimate response to disability, but we have no evidence on the differences between men and women in response to spinal injury. Socioeconomic status has been implicated as a factor in outcome in one study, but not enough is known about its role at this point. It and culture may have very powerful influences on adjustment to spinal injury since these environment variables relate to resources available and expectations regarding behavior. Both of these latter issues may interfere with the rehabilitation process. The factor of urban versus rural residence was implicated in one study of marriage and spinal injury, but no conclusions can be drawn at this time. Thus, much research needs to be done on the influence of demographic variables on adjustment to spinal injury.

Rehabilitation personnel are often asked to rate the behavior of the person with a disability, but there is considerable evidence to demonstrate that they consistently overestimate the degree of psychological distress present. In addition, there is some evidence to suggest that many personnel may have an unrealistic stereotype of the disabled person which is not very different from that of the general population. Since these rehabilitation personnel form part of the patient's environment, these expectations as to how disabled people should behave may be counterproductive influences at a time when the person's self-image is most vulnerable.

There is no evidence of a unitary spinal cord injury personality. In fact, there is considerable evidence to suggest that the population of persons with spinal injury is a heterogeneous one, and thus it is fallacious to attempt to describe the average person. Very few persons display significant psychopathology after the spinal injury unless they had a preinjury history of hospitalization for depression or suicide attempts or other evidence of severe maladjustment. There are clinical reports that psychotic persons who sustain a spinal injury may show a remission of the psychotic symptoms until pressured to leave the hospital and resume function in the outside world.

The research into the factors associated with adjustment to spinal injury suggests that youth, a warm and loving family background, financial resources, a history of accepting responsibility for educational and vocational plans, an internal locus of control, interpersonal support, creativity in problem solving, having many goals, and goals in the accomplishment versus physical function area are associated with success. However, most of the research has focused on features of the person exclusively rather than on person-environment units. In addition, such research activity tends to identify the successes so that we can screen out the failures. However, this assumes that all responsibility for success depends on the intrinsic characteristics of the person, and suggestions are not given as to how to deal with the failures. This limited approach may be too costly if the death rate from self-neglect is viewed as one indication of the problem.

The use of psychological tests to predict outcome has not been the focus of much research, but in cases in which they have been used, they have not accounted for much of the variance in behavior. Rather, direct observation of the behavior in question is a more powerful predictor of future behavior. The Minnesota Multiphasic Personality Inventory (MMPI) has been used to assess immediate response to spinal injury and only mild depression has been found. However, there is the implicit assumption of homogeneity of the population with spinal injury and that assumption is probably erroneous. The population seems to be very heterogeneous and may be composed of several distinct groups. Therefore, the averaging of psychological test data for the entire group, before the nature of the population has been determined, may produce misleading results. Furthermore, the MMPI, for example, has been found to contain items that a person with spinal injury would have to answer in the deviant direction, not because of psychological problems but because of the spinal injury. This inflates the profiles spuriously unless a correction is made for these items.

No data exists relating the results of intelligence tests or projective tests to outcome. However, there is some evidence to suggest that tests of creativity and problem-solving ability may relate to outcome. Therefore, it is recommended that psychological test data be considered to be only one of many kinds of measurements of behavior. Greater emphasis should be given to the direct observation of behavior in our evaluation and research activity.

Although rehabilitation has traditionally focused on the physical parameters of the disability, the social implications of the disability may be devastating and should receive equal attention in our rehabilitation programs. The concept of difference is learned at an early age, as is the concept of physical attractiveness, and we learn to evaluate people on these two dimensions. Thus, the person with spinal injury may devalue himself according to these standards that he himself learned, and he knows that others will devalue him accordingly. As a result, the person with spinal injury tends to withdraw from most social situations after discharge from the rehabilitation center. Through a process of self-socialization a person learns to cope with his world to some degree, and there is great variability among people as to the degree of skill they achieve in managing social situations. It appears that a key to a successful outcome after spinal injury is social skills. Therefore, a major emphasis for the future must be the development of techniques to teach social skills and the implementation of research to identify which technique is best suited to which behavioral goal.

Disability can have a great impact on the family, but there is no data to document the types of problems and the intervention strategies that are most effective as remedial devices. Statistics on marriage and divorce among United States veterans suggest that approximately 26 percent of preinjury and postinjury marriages end in divorce. However, one study of marriages among civilians with spinal injury indicated that marriages contracted preinjury were exceedingly vulnerable to dissolution in comparison to marriages contracted after injury. This was particularly true for women with spinal injury.

Recreation has often been viewed as a luxury, merely an entertainment, rather than a therapeutic activity. However, it appears that active participation in a sport may have physical and psychosocial benefits that should be studied. Since recreation of some kind is an important part of everyone's life, a person with a disability needs to learn new leisure time activities if his preinjury ones are no longer available. The effects of active participation in sports and recreational activity should be studied in terms of productivity and in terms of the death rate.

Traditionally, there has been an emphasis on full-time employment as *the* outcome of rehabilitation efforts. However, employment may not be an appropriate goal for everyone, and there are obstacles within the economic system that prevent everyone who desires a job from becoming employed. Therefore, it seems more reasonable to consider productivity to be the goal, which includes educational and avocational activities, group membership, family and community participation, in addition to employment.

The data suggest that persons with paraplegia are somewhat more likely to obtain employment than persons with quadriplegia. Yet the employment rate varies from 14 percent to 44 percent depending upon the definitions of employment. Obstacles to employment include the financial disincentives to productivity, negative attitudes of employers, and lack of complete services by departments of rehabilitation. As with psychological factors, the research tends to focus exclusively on the characteristics of the person that lead to success. The emphasis is on the identification of winners and the attempt to screen out the losers rather than on the development of strategies that will identify marketable skills, train these skills, and place the person in a job that utilizes these skills. However, unless the financial disincentives to productivity are reduced, many persons with disabilities will not be able to afford to take a job even though they would like to work.

In addition, as with social attitudes, a huge program to educate the public or employers is not recommended as a means of reducing prejudice toward the disabled. Rather, we should devote our efforts to teaching the disabled to function successfully in the able-bodied world. This will require able-bodied people to interact with those with disabilities and to behave in a normal, nonprejudicial manner. As people change their behavior toward disabled persons, their cognitions and emotions will gradually change over time. Thus, an emphasis on behavior change as a means of producing attitude change is recommended rather than the reverse.

Sexual function is an important part of life and continues following spinal injury. There is some evidence to suggest that the sex drive may be slightly reduced following spinal injury, but age variables may play a powerful role. Evidence suggests that persons who abstain from sexual activities are no less well adjusted than those who participate. However, whether one participates in sexual activities seems to be highly dependent on having a partner with whom a good relationship exists. In fact, within successful marriages, a significant proportion of the couples do not rely on sexual intercourse as their primary mode of sexual satisfaction. Thus, sexual function has many parameters that need to be evaluated and methods of relating sexually need to be taught. Each person with spinal injury should have the opportunity to participate in a sexual relationship if he or she chooses; thus, training should be offered.

However, the treatments for sexual dysfunctions, judging by the literature, seem to consist of counseling-didactic sessions and sexual attitude readjustment workshops. There is no evidence that these techniques lead to behavior change on the part of the participants, although most participants report that the sessions are helpful. Therefore, strategies for teaching people a variety of sexual behaviors need to be developed, and the outcome of these efforts must be studied. There are no data on the effect of disability on the partner nor strategies to assist partners to cope with the disability. Much research is needed in this area.

The treatment environment—the hospital or rehabilitation center—seems to have a profound effect on the behavior of the person with the disability. Evidence suggests that the hospital environment provides minimal opportunity for patient decision making, independence, or zest in any of the treatment activities that comprise a large part of rehabilitation. In fact, the treatment environment accounts for more variability in patient behavior than individual patient characteristics do. In addition, there is evidence that a large part of a patient's day is spent in nontherapeutic activities and alone. Aides and orderlies are the personnel who have most patient contact, but they receive the least training in behavior change skills. Thus, patients are rewarded for dependent, nonassertive behaviors and ignored when they try to be independent. As a result, the rehabilitation process must be studied to determine its effect on patient behavior and to determine if that is the effect we desire. If not, then either we must change the procedures of rehabilitation centers, or we must develop a multistage rehabilitation system: physical rehabilitation followed by training in functional skills for living.

There is considerable discussion in the literature about the importance of individual counseling, group counseling, and psychotherapy as treatment techniques following onset of disability. However, there is no evidence to demonstrate that these techniques lead to improved functioning and behavior change. It is apparent that many of the goals are too globally defined, impossible to measure, and, perhaps, inappropriate for the technique in question.

Thus, it is time to perform some carefully controlled studies to assess the effectiveness of counseling techniques as behavior change strategies.

Behavior therapy has been demonstrated to lead to behavior change in fluid intake, pushups, body positioning in bed, personal hygiene, and upper extremity strengthening. By using such techniques, "unmotivated" persons can achieve similar levels of function to the "motivated" person. Since all of rehabilitation is a learning process, a behavior change process, intervention strategies must be evaluated for their ability to produce behavior change. Behavior therapy techniques are ones that have demonstrated this effect. In addition, if most behavior is learned through the principles of operant conditioning, then behavior therapy techniques should become the standard operating procedure of rehabilitation and all personnel should become skilled in such strategies.

Social skills training shows promise as an intervention strategy, but there is only one research project that has studied its effect on behavior change in persons with spinal injury. Development of social skills training strategies should be a primary focus of research along with the study of which types of settings are most appropriate for use of such techniques.

Because of the counterproductive effect of present hospital environments on patient behavior, alternative methods of service delivery must be studied. The transitional living center concept shows promise and should be studied further. We must consider the possibility of a multistage rehabilitation process and study the cost effectiveness of such an approach. Furthermore, since a minority of new spinal injuries each year receive treatment through one of the regional spinal injury centers, other methods for the delivery of services should be studied. The case manager approach and homebound rehabilitation programs are among the alternatives that show promise. Independent living centers may be an additional resource within the community and deserve to be studied.

Basically, the emphasis in rehabilitation should shift from physical functioning to psychosocial integration into the community. The latter entails the former, but the reverse is not true. To accomplish this, we need to expand the content of rehabilitation programs to include social and productivity skills training in addition to ADL and mobility training. We need to change our model of rehabilitation service delivery from a medical model to a learning model. We need to shift our research emphasis from the identification of winners and losers (the study of person variables exclusively) to the development of behavior change strategies to help people with spinal injury cope with their own world (the study of the person-environment interaction). Finally, to assess the utility of these changes, we need to execute carefully controlled research that will specify behavioral outcomes and use direct measurements of behavior.

Part III

Future Directions

10
Research Issues and Methodologies

THE NEED FOR RESEARCH

Our search for knowledge is imperfect and the information that is transmitted from one person to another is always tempered by elements of personal interpretation and acts of judgment. Through research endeavors of various kinds, some experimentally controlled and some entailing naturalistic observations, professionals can increase the amount of information about which persons agree despite vagaries of interpretation and judgment. Research should be impartial and unbiased, a goal of science not always achieved, however (Barber 1976).

Within the field of spinal cord injury, research into the physiological and mechanical aspects of injury, treatment, and maintenance has proceeded rapidly. But research into the psychological, social, and vocational parameters of life after spinal injury seems to have been stalemated. This is partly because of the difficulty in conducting research using "soft" data, the low value that has been placed on such research by funding agencies and administrators of rehabilitation centers, and the lack of adequately trained research personnel to initiate and carry out the projects. If progress is to be made, the last two elements must change. The first element need not be a deterrent given the necessary funding and manpower.

There are at least four reasons for conducting research: to assess the outcomes of rehabilitation programs; to assess the effects of different treatment strategies; to separate the promising candidates from the less promising ones; and to study the rehabilitation process.

"Accountability is the watchword—evaluation is the handmaiden. More and more there will be an emphasis on producing results" (Garrett 1976, p. 96). In the past, it was acceptable to agree that rehabilitation was "good," and as long as the efforts were well-intentioned, the results were assumed to be good also. If outcomes were assessed, the assessment was performed sporadically and often by the very person who designed the program and implemented the treatment approach, hardly an impartial analysis. Furthermore, the definition of outcome would vary from one study to another and frequently was stated in terms of an abstract concept (adjustment, success) that could not be directly measured but only inferred and judged by a rater. Therefore, it has been impossible to compare the results of one study with another.

Research utilizing outcomes such as "adjustment," "success," and "rehabilitated," as the item to be measured will be flawed and difficult to interpret. Each of these terms is an abstract concept that cannot be measured directly. The concept of adjustment, for example, can only be *inferred* by measuring the multitude of component behaviors encompassed by the concept of adjustment. However, customarily in research the component behaviors of adjustment are not specified, are not measured, and the concept of adjustment will be rated in global, nonspecific terms.

Furthermore, there is no agreement as to the proper outcome of our rehabilitation efforts. Attainment of full-time employment for 60 days has been one outcome identified in a number of studies, but there is growing concern that such an indicator may have limited utility (Professional Conference 1977). Therefore, to avoid compounding the errors of judgment and interpretation, the *behavior* of the person with spinal injury must be assessed in units that are observable and enumerable. Once a large amount of data is amassed describing what people with spinal injury actually do following their rehabilitation programs, we can begin to determine which of these behaviors constitute success or adjustment. If we assess behavior, we have the basis for being able to compare the data from many studies and to begin to evaluate the effects of our rehabilitation efforts. There are two projects, currently in progress, that hope to provide a methodology for assessing outcomes in behavioral terms: the Rehabilitation Indicators Project (Diller, Fordyce, Jacobs, and Brown 1977) and the Longitudinal Functional Assessment System (Willems 1976b). These will be discussed later in this chapter.

A second purpose for doing research is to assess the effects of different treatment strategies. This should be one of the major foci for the future. There are a large number of new techniques available that have some demonstrated utility as behavior change strategies and may be very useful within rehabilitation. Some techniques may be more effective in achieving certain behavioral outcomes than others, and certain persons may function better using some strategies than others. Thus, research will be necessary to define the parameters of this matrix of person variables, treatment variables, and outcome variables. Good research of this type could lead to dramatic advances in the state of the art and should be emphasized in the future. The outcomes of such research must be defined in *behavioral* terms, units that can be observed and counted, if progress is going to be made in this area.

Traditionally, research into the psychological, social, and vocational aspects of spinal injury has focused on the attempt to separate the promising from less promising candidates for rehabilitation. This is the third purpose for conducting research. Most of the literature reviewed in this document has been of this nature, and the emphasis has been on the assets and liabilities of the person that lead to success or failure (person variables exclusively). Implicit in each of these studies is the assumption that the person has the major share of the responsibility for becoming a success. All he had to do was to cooperate with the rehabilitation program which was assumed to be a ''good'' one. If the person failed and did not become a success, it was because of flaws in his character labeled variously as poor motivation, denial of disability, or not having adjusted to the disability.

The person does have a responsibility for his future as a disabled person and must accept responsibility for his own life, but this is not the only factor in the equation leading to success $[B = f(P \times O \times E)]$. If the person succeeds, then it is assumed to be the result of a ''good'' rehabilitation program. But if the person fails, then it is because of flaws in his character. Not so. Our programs are fallible and often do not assist the person with a spinal injury to achieve goals that relate to survival outside of the hospital. There is considerable evidence that the environment has a tremendous influence on the disabled person's behavior. Vash (Professional Conference 1977) refers to the distal and proximal environmental influences. The proximal environment consists of the treatment and social environment, the immediate physical environment, and distal refers to welfare legislation, financial disincentives to productivity, and employer attitudes. The literature provides some evidence and considerable opinion about the effects of both of these environments on the behavior of the person with spinal injury. This, then, raises the question, what is a less promising candidate? Is it a person with severe character flaws, is it a person whose environment is full of obstacles, or is it a combination of both factors?

Promising candidate research is not unimportant, but it is a lower priority in comparison to some of the other research needs. In addition, if the behavior of the person with spinal injury is documented while in the rehabilitation program and over the years, a data base will be formed that will permit us to assess outcomes. If multiple approaches to treatment are utilized with each person, the less promising candidate will be the person for whom nothing works. The definition then becomes an empirical one.

The literature has defined the successful rehabilitation candidate as young, with a good, loving family background, without significant psychological problems, and who has a history of educational and vocational planning and accomplishment. One might hypothesize that these persons account for 20 percent of the total and that they might succeed even without our rehabilitation program. They have the outstanding personal characteristics that allow them to overcome the environmental obstacles confronting a disabled person. Perhaps another 20 percent are labeled as poor rehabilitation candidates because they have such a poor history of coping with life and an environment full of so many obstacles that the probability of their living a trouble-free life as a person with spinal injury is slim. The middle 60 percent of the spinal cord injury population could be described as the average person, who is not outstanding in either talents or environmental supports, and who finds the onset of spinal injury to be a very significant challenge in his or her ability to cope.

Using the traditional approach, which focuses on the person as the sole factor responsible for successful outcome, there will be a success rate of 20 percent who will become financially independent through competitive employment under present circumstances. It is hypothesized that 80 percent would not succeed with this approach.

However, if environmental modifications and alternate treatment strategies did lead to behavior change on the part of the person, and if *each* person were approached in terms of the strategies that could be used to assist him to cope with his environment, then the behaviors needed could be identified and the strategies that are best suited to that behavior change situation would be utilized. As a result, the progress of the 20 percent who might have succeeded anyway would be facilitated, and the level of functioning of the 60 percent who are average may be improved. This could lead to a success rate of 80 percent. Those whose level of functioning remains problematical will be identified in an empirical manner and may account for 20 percent or less of the total population with spinal injury. Thus, using the promising candidate approach, the success rate may be 20 percent; using the multiple treatment strategy approach, the success rate might approach 80 percent. This is a hypothetical situation, and some might criticize that the philosophy of rehabilitation is being confused with strategy for research. However, the two are highly correlated since the philosophy of rehabilitation will define what questions become researched.

The literature suggests that research into the identification of promising candidates has not been very productive. Rather, it is the person in interaction with his environment that is the critical feature of all rehabilitation efforts. Therefore, *to change the person's behavior, the environment must be modified;* thus, research into person-environment interactions and strategies to modify these interactions seems to be the key to future progress in rehabilitation.

A fourth purpose for research is to study rehabilitation as a process, as a highly complex system of interacting elements that evolves over time. If we accept the premise that the critical need is to evaluate different treatment strategies, then we have to study the rehabilitation center from an ecological point of view. The physical structure, the staffing pattern, and the organizational policies are facets of the environment that influence the behavior of the person with spinal injury. If our research focus is to identify those factors influencing the behavior of the person with spinal injury, then the environment in which the treatment is delivered must be studied. In addition, it will be important to identify the impact of different treatment environments —alternative models of rehabilitation service delivery—on different classes of behavior.

THE FOCUS OF MEASUREMENT

A large number of the studies have attempted to define the factors associated with adjustment to disability or success following spinal injury. However, there is not a consensus as to what constitutes adjustment or success. In addition, the methodology of assessing these criteria was frequently the ratings of rehabilitation staff, often without specification as to the behaviors of the patient that were being rated.

Athelstan and Crewe (1977) believe that there are multiple dimensions to adjustment which they are attempting to define. However, it is difficult to define adjustment in terms that are applicable to all persons with spinal injury and in terms that do not involve value judgments. Trieschmann (1971, 1974) proposed that success or adjustment to spinal injury might include at least three dimensions:

1. Prevention of medical complications and performance of the ADL and mobility skills that are practical given the person's living circumstances.
2. Maintenance of a stable living environment.
3. Productivity (social, family, recreational, community, and vocational activities).

Within each of these dimensions, specific behavioral goals could be determined, and a goal attainment scaling procedure (Kiresuk and Sherman 1968; Kiresuk 1973) could be used to assess success. Thus, within each of these categories behavioral goals might be set relating to the person's unique combination of circumstances. Use of this technique would allow one to measure the success with which a program assisted the person in achieving his goals, and yet the definition of adjustment could vary across persons depending on their unique combination of circumstances.

Another focus for research is to identify psychological traits within the person. Self-concept, self-esteem, and locus of control are psychological traits that may be factors in coping with spinal injury. However, they cannot be measured directly, since they are abstract concepts. Rather, the presence of a positive self-concept, for example, is inferred from a large number of verbal and motor behaviors that the person displays. Although self-concept cannot be measured directly, these verbal and motor behaviors can be measured and, in aggregate, the self-concept can be estimated.

However, some of the psychological tests or rating scales used in many research projects that have been designed to measure self-concept, for example, will measure the verbal behavior of the person to that test stimulus only. The correlation of that test behavior to the large number of other behaviors encompassed by the abstraction *self-concept* is usually not reported (and usually has not been demonstrated). Thus, there is a problem. Too many studies have purported to evaluate abstract concepts without the proper methodology or understanding to do so.

Another focus of measurement efforts is the actual behavior of the person with the disability. Verbal and motor behaviors that are observable and quantifiable can be identified and should be the focus of our studies. We must differentiate between the behavior that the person *can do* and the behavior that the person *does do*. Too often, this differentiation is not made, and, therefore, many ADL and mobility assessment procedures rate what the patient can do. However, Willems (1976a) has found that there is a low correlation between ratings of capacity (what the person can do) and the behavior that actually does occur when the person is in his own environment. Sand, Fordyce, and Fowler (1973) conclude that the best predictor of future fluid intake behavior is not the battery of psychological tests but the actual fluid intake behavior in the first two weeks in the rehabilitation center. They recommend that rather than focusing on trying to predict who will behave in what fashion, we should measure the behavior in question and then apply strategies to shape the behavior to the desired level.

A fourth focus for measurements is the behavior of the rehabilitation staff. In the study of the environment and rehabilitation process, it is important to measure, not only the patients' behavior, but the behavior of the staff also. The study by Mikulic (1971) is an important example of this approach. Marr, Greenwood, and Roessler (1977) are conducting a research project that will provide a behavioral analysis of a rehabilitation service delivery system. They will meet with clients and service delivery personnel in order to identify problems in giving and receiving service. The antecedents of the problem are identified, along with the behaviors and the consequences. Through an innovative approach such as this we may be able to identify ways to improve the efficiency with which we can teach persons with spinal injury to cope with the disability. However, in order to do this, we, rehabilitation personnel, must be willing to examine our own behavior rather than restricting our focus exclusively to the behavior of the person with a disability.

However, since the purpose of rehabilitation is to assist the person in developing a repertoire of behaviors which are effective in dealing with the world, the focus of our measurements must be this repertoire of behaviors. Therefore, the various measurement methodologies must be examined to determine their adequacy in giving us the information needed: What does the person actually do?

METHODS OF MEASUREMENT

Self-ratings

Many studies have used the self-ratings of the person with the disability as either the single method of measurement or in conjunction with other measures. In each case, what is being measured is the person's verbal behavior.

Whether or not this verbal behavior is the purported focus of the study varies, but often it is not. Frequently, the purpose of a study may be to study the effect of spinal injury on feelings of depression or the effect of group therapy on self-concept, for example. However, the validity of the self-rating as a measure of depression or self-concept is usually not reported because the researcher is satisfied with face validity.

Self-ratings may be very useful in research as one of many measures of an outcome, as in Lawson's (1976, 1978) study of depression after spinal injury. Self-ratings may be useful if the purpose of the study is to assess the effects of a treatment on self-ratings per se. However, if generalizations of the data from self-ratings are made, then evidence should be provided that such generalizations are appropriate. In an era of accountability, interest in evaluation has increased and self-ratings are often used as a substitute for other more complex but less readily available measures. Yet, if progress is going to be made in our efforts to increase our knowledge about the effects of spinal injury, more sophisticated and appropriate measures of the intended effect will have to be used.

Self-reports through Interview or Questionnaire

The validity of self-report measures has been a concern to scientists for many years (Webb, Campbell, Schwartz, and Sechrest 1966; Franklin and Osborne 1971) and should be of greater concern to researchers in rehabilitation than it has apparently been. Both methods may be very helpful in the collection of demographic data, but the detail of the data obtained may vary across subjects because of the highly structured and often restricted nature of the questionnaires and the variability in the interactions between interviewer and subject. Many studies have described the adjustment to disability based on judgments made by the interviewer who was also the designer of the experiment or project. The opportunity for bias is overwhelming and difficult to assess (Barber 1976). In the Kemp and Vash (1971) study, the data were obtained through a structured interview conducted by one of the researchers, but judgments based on that interview data were made independently by another group of professionals, thus reducing the opportunity for bias.

Questionnaire and interview studies have the additional problems of self-selection of the subjects and the degree of cooperation in complying with the researcher's requests. This is a problem in many follow-up studies, as noted by Felton and Litman (1965) and Grynbaum and associates (1963). It is not known how the sample that chooses to respond to a mailed questionnaire or to participate in a study differs from the sample that does not participate. In addition, there is concern that in questionnaire studies, the more successful group chooses to respond, whereas in interview studies for follow-up purposes, those who make themselves available may have problems that need attention. Those who are successful often are too busy to give the time necessary to come back for an evaluation. These problems do exist and can never be completely eliminated, but attempts should be made to control for them. An unbiased interviewer is essential, and efforts should be made to obtain a representative sample of the population. The follow-up through the National Spinal Cord Injury Data Research Center will be helpful, but there are concerns about the representativeness of its sample (Professional Conference 1977).

A major problem that interview and questionnaire techniques share is the delimited nature of the data that they collect. The person, at one specific moment in time, is asked to describe his behavior which flows and evolves over time. Rates of behavior and contingencies can only be estimated and depend largely on the accuracy and cooperation of the subject. Data that are very important to an understanding of the person's behavior may not be collected unless it is part of the questionnaire or interview. Thus, information gained through these techniques may not be truly representative of what the person actually does.

Diaries

One method for obtaining a representative sample of the flow of a person's behavior is to have him keep a diary of everything he does. The problem of inaccuracy because of poor cooperation remains, but inaccuracy because of errors in recall or estimation has been largely eliminated. This method has been used very successfully by Fordyce and associates (1973) and Fordyce (1976) in the management of patients with chronic pain. In addition, Willems (1976a, 1976b) has been using this technique and has found it to be promising.

Although the advantage of this method is its representativeness of the actual flow of behavior over time in each person's unique fashion, a disadvantage is the need to categorize the data in some manner in order to summarize the behavior of one person over time or to compare the behaviors of many people. To use this method adequately, systems for reporting and comparing the data in standardized terms will have to be developed.

Telephone Interviews

Widmer (1978) has studied a method of obtaining a descriptive log of ongoing daily behaviors out in the community in contrast to tallying the frequencies of a few targeted behaviors. On a sample of persons with spinal injury who were keeping a diary of daily activities, a random telephone interview schedule was implemented to assess the validity of information gained in 20 minutes. Data gathered by telephone correlated highly with diaries of daily activities. This method seems to be a practical and reliable way to gather behavioral data from persons in their home and community environments over fairly long periods of time. The advantages of this method are that the responsibility for the data collection is placed on the researcher, not the subject, and what the person actually does do over time in his own environment is measured.

Staff Ratings

Staff ratings of patient behavior are the foundation of many ADL and mobility assessments, and this method has been applied to issues in psychosocial research as well. However, the evidence suggests that rehabilitation staff are notoriously inaccurate when asked to rate the presence or degree of a psychological trait in their patients. The evidence provided by Taylor (1967) has been duplicated in many studies. Rehabilitation staff consistently overestimate the degree of psychological distress in their patients. In addition, Albrecht and Higgins (1977) compared multiple measures of success in a rehabilitation center and found that the intercorrelations of staff ratings of patient adjustment, self-ratings by patients, and psychological test scores were very low.

The problem with staff ratings of psychological processes occurs in part because of the staff's lack of training in assessment of these factors but more particularly because of the nature of the task itself. The psychological traits that the staff are asked to rate are abstract concepts that cannot be measured directly. Rather, these traits are composed of many individual behaviors which, as an aggregate, are described by the summary term, the psychological trait label. Thus, the staff have been asked to do a task for which they have not been trained, and the component behaviors of the trait are usually not specified.

Biochemical Measures of Emotion

Measurement of emotions is a methodologically difficult problem. Hohmann (1966) reports that emotions may be experienced at a cognitive level and less at a physiological level after spinal injury. Rehabilitation staff consistently overestimate the presence of emotions in their patients. And patient self-reports may be influenced by staff expectations that they should be very emotional about their disability; thus, Hohmann reports that many patients act "as if" they were feeling emotional. Biochemical measures may therefore be very helpful in any study that purports to assess emotional reactions following spinal cord injury.

Lawson's study (1976, 1978) of depression can serve as a model of the multiple levels of measurement that are necessary to document many psychological processes. Not only did he use two types of measures of the patients' verbal behavior to assess depression, but he used staff ratings and a biochemical measure as well. In addition, all of his measures were made daily over an extended period of time. As a result, he had a large data base which allowed him to determine empirically at what points in the hospitalization depression occurred and for how long, rather than predetermining which incidents should be emotion producing and taking segmental measures of emotion, as in the study conducted by McDaniel and Sexton (1970). In their study they chose four incidents and obtained biochemical measures at each of the four times, and, as a result, their data are very difficult to interpret.

Thus, there are two issues that must be considered in studies of emotional reactions to disability. We need multiple measures of emotion, including a biochemical one, and we need longitudinal data rather than cross-sectional data. The demands of this kind of research are great, but it appears to be a waste of time and money to compromise on these issues.

Direct Observations

One of the best predictors of future behavior is the rate at which the behavior is occurring now. This was noted in the study of fluid intake behavior by Sand and associates (1973), and it has been a core principle of psychology. So many of the behaviors that are the focus of our rehabilitation efforts can be observed and counted, and, thus, it is perplexing that this methodology is used so infrequently. By defining the behavior in question and then counting its frequency of occurrence, progress can be assessed and programs planned to increase or decrease these rates. And by counting behaviors, a strategy becomes available to assess the psychological traits that have traditionally been so important.

For example, Vineberg and Willems (1971) wanted to measure independence. This was defined as initiation of the behavior by the patient. Thus they counted the number of behaviors initiated by that patient and compared this to the total number of behaviors performed. As a result, they could assess the development of independence over time and in different hospital settings. Zest (or motivation) was defined as the initiation of a behavior and the active participation in the behavior, and was measured in a similar fashion. Lawson (1976, 1978) used rate of speech during the first three minutes of a tape recording of the daily events as one of his measures of depression (i.e., the number of words spoken in three minutes). Consequently, many of the components of rehabilitation can be defined operationally and counted.

The behavior sample technique, which can be helpful in vocational planning, is a related methodology and may be very helpful in research on social skills training, for example. The ultimate test of the effectiveness of assertiveness training and social skills training is changes in behavior in actual social situations, not changes on a paper-pencil test. Therefore, the behavior sample technique may be most helpful in assessing the outcomes of such programs.

Mechanical Measures of Behavior

Certain behaviors are capable of being monitored by mechanical devices thus reducing the cost of assessment procedures. Halstead (1973, 1976) has described the use of unobstructive monitoring devices, such as a wheelchair odometer and the rest-time monitor. The wheelchair odometer provides one measure of activity and increasing rates of activity in the initial rehabilitation phase can be one measure of progress. Frieden and Halstead (1976) describe the use of the wheelchair odometer in a noninstitutional setting; they found that 5–15 miles per week may be the average for an independent person following spinal injury. Vash (Professional Conference 1977), however, cautions against the setting of standards of distance traveled as a measure of productivity since, for some persons or types of tasks, high rates of distance traveled in a wheelchair may signify low productivity. Frieden and Halstead have recognized this problem and describe it as "spinning one's wheels."

The rest-time monitor consists of pressure sensitive pads which, when connected to a recording device, can give measures of time in and out of bed. This device, along with the wheelchair odometer, are examples of mechanical devices that can provide important information to rehabilitation programs about patient progress and that can help to solve the problem of how to measure behavior outside of the institutional setting. Devices such as this should be developed and tested since they help focus on that most important issue: What the person actually does do over time.

Behavioral Mapping

Miller and Keith (1973) have demonstrated the utility of behavioral mapping as a technique for assessing the behavior of a system, such as a rehabilitation center. A behavioral map involves the recording of the physical location of inhabitants at various times and a system of categorization of their activity. The results of behavioral mapping yield information on the types of activity that occur in various locations at various times. Such information can indicate the density of inhabitants per space, the extent of usage of areas, whether areas encourage multiple or single activities, the flow of inhabitants from area to area, the proportion of a study population engaged in an activity at any one time, and other kinds of data. Miller and Keith note that an important feature of this technique is its assessment of actual behaviors in rehabilitation centers versus assumptions about what happens in a rehabilitation center.

Study of the rehabilitation process will be necessary in order to identify programs that work versus those that are less effective. Techniques such as behavioral mapping are one measure of how rehabilitation centers function. Even though such assessment can be very threatening to the administrators and personnel in such centers, we must begin to look carefully at what we are doing and its effect on our patients. If we are afraid of such assessment procedures and the results, then we should ask ourselves why.

Environmental Negotiability Survey

The hospital environment has been carefully modified to facilitate the behaviors of disabled persons. This masks the extent to which a disabled person's ability to perform a task may vary in other environments. Thus, measures of ADL and mobility skills within the hospital may correlate poorly with actual behavior in one's own environment (Willems 1976a), which is the true measure of outcome of rehabilitation programs. For this reason, Norris-Baker (1978) has developed and tested an environmental negotiability survey. The concept of negotiability emphasizes the person's ability to interact with the physical features of his own environment. Thus, this is one of the only true measures of the behavior-environment interaction.

The environmental negotiability survey has two parts, the environmental inventory and the negotiability assessment. For the first part, a trained rater lists all of the objects in the person's home environment that are visible and require some kind of behavior in their use. Any objects that might limit the person's mobility are listed. For the second part, the rater and the disabled person tour the home together and the rater makes a yes/no decision about the person's ability to use every object on the inventory list. The focus is on whether or not the person, with only his usual assistive equipment, can actually use the object independently for its normal purpose. It is interesting to note that raters' predictions of whether or not the person could use the object were significantly less accurate in comparison with the person's actual behavior with the object.

This survey reflects progress over time in the proportion of objects that are negotiable. Home modifications, environment changes, and the utility of various assistive devices (such as, electric wheelchair) can be assessed. In combination with the telephone interview, the environmental negotiability survey provides direct measures of actual behavior in one's own environment. Thus, the opportunity to gather meaningful outcome data is available.

Psychological Tests

The review of the literature in chapter 3 did not reveal a single psychological test that has been demonstrated to be a powerful predictor of ability to function successfully following spinal cord injury. There is evidence that tests of creativity and problem-solving ability are one of the several variables that correlate with productivity (Kemp and Vash 1971), but there have not been many predictive studies using these psychological tests in spinal injury.

When psychological tests are used as measurement devices, certain precautions should be considered. Very few tests have norms for disabled persons, particularly persons with spinal cord injury. Taylor (1967, 1970) discovered that a person with spinal cord injury will respond to a certain number of items on the Minnesota Multiphasic Personality Inventory (MMPI) in the scorable direction considered pathological, not because of psychological maladjustments but because of the spinal injury. Thus, the MMPI profiles of persons with spinal injury will be spuriously inflated unless corrected for these items. Although the MMPI has the most extensive developmental history of almost all psychological tests (except for the Wechsler tests, Stanford-Binet, and Strong Vocational Interest Blank), and norms were obtained for persons with legitimate medical disorders, this error in the profiles of persons with spinal injury was detected only relatively recently in the history of the test. Thus, professionals should be cautious in the use of psychological tests and not use them as the primary measure of the behavior of the person after spinal injury. Direct observation of behavior is very important.

The use of intelligence tests with persons with spinal injury entails all of the considerations that are relevant to other populations. The relationship between the Verbal IQ on the Wechsler Adult Intelligence Scale (WAIS) and functioning following spinal injury has not been demonstrated, and its usefulness in predicting vocational achievement needs to be tested. The use of the performance scales with persons with impaired hand function is inappropriate, and warnings about this should be introduced into the test manual. All of the norms for the performance items, except picture completion, were based on unimpaired hand function. Thus, perceptual motor intelligence cannot be assessed readily in persons with quadriplegia.

Scales measuring locus of control show some evidence of being predictive of those behaviors associated with success following spinal injury. Therefore, in research efforts, professionals should consider a variety of measurement options, psychological tests being only one of many.

In summary, there is no one measurement that is perfect; each has advantages and disadvantages. Behavior is very complex and, in the future, professionals should attempt to measure this complexity by using multiple levels of measurement of the behavior in question. The studies reviewed in this document reveal the tremendous amount of wasted effort that occurs when professionals do not carefully identify the behavioral issue they are studying and do not select the types of measurement techniques that will appropriately and accurately assess the effects they hope to study. More productive research endeavors will require a focus on observable and countable behaviors and the use of measurement techniques that will provide such data. Development of mechanical measurement devices that are unobtrusive should be given great emphasis, as should the implementation of measurement strategies that document the daily behaviors occurring in rehabilitation centers on the part of patients and staff. Use of such measurement strategies in the home environment will be essential.

METHODOLOGICAL ISSUES IN FUTURE RESEARCH

There are several methodological issues that must be considered in future research in spinal cord injury if such future efforts expect to advance the state of the art. Greater care must be taken in the selection of a sample for a study than has been taken in the past. Evidence suggests that the population of persons with spinal cord injury is heterogeneous, but homogeneity has been assumed in most studies. Sample characteristics should be documented and studied in a controlled fashion.

The representativeness of a sample should be examined more thoroughly than in the past. Follow-up studies must make greater efforts to locate the entire group under consideration and to assess the influence of the self-selection factors discussed earlier.

In addition, studies using the population of persons treated at regional spinal cord injury centers may be biased since less than 15 percent of the national population of persons with spinal injury come into contact with such centers. Therefore, data must be obtained on persons treated outside of the regional system for comparison purposes. Efforts should be made to include a sample of nonregional system persons in any follow-up sponsored by the Rehabilitation Services Administration. Either this data should be included in the National Spinal Cord Injury Data Research Center data base, or a separate study should be conducted that would seek out and study a sample that is representative of the nation.

Studies assessing treatment effects should use random assignment of cases, and control groups should be employed. The basic principles of accepted research design should be utilized.

The measures employed in research should include the direct observations of the behavior under study or instruments that have documented reliability and criterion validity. Paper and pencil tests and rating scales, if created for the project, should demonstrate their correlation with the particular behavior under study on samples other than the one used in the research.

Multiple levels of measurement should be used whenever possible, especially when the focus of the study is a psychological trait or emotional reaction. Longitudinal research should be emphasized because learning to live with a disability is a dynamic process and not a static event. Furthermore, behavior-environment units should be the focus of research since evidence suggests that environments may account for more variance in behavior than we have recognized. Measurement systems must be developed that can provide a standardized system for the assessment of outcomes. With the advent of such systems, there will be greater opportunity to compare the results of one study with those of another.

TWO APPROACHES TO OUTCOME MEASUREMENT

There are two projects currently in progress that address the issue of outcome measurement in behavioral terms: The Rehabilitation Indicators Project (Diller, Fordyce, Jacobs, and Brown 1977) and the Longitudinal Functional Assessment System (Willems 1976b). Each shows promise of advancing the state of the art of measurement in rehabilitation.

The Rehabilitation Indicators Project (RIP) has focused on developing a lexicon of behaviors that will define the behavioral domain relevant to rehabilitation efforts. There are status indicators, such as employed versus unemployed, marital status, etc. There are activity pattern indicators, such as cleaning house, going to work, telephoning friends. In addition, there are skill indicators, such as using a knife and fork to eat, dressing oneself, and others. Environment indicators will be developed to assess features of the person's environment relevant to function. So far the lexicon includes 10 status items, 50 activity patterns, 450 skill indicators, and the environment indicators are being developed.

This lexicon will provide a compendium of specific behaviors that may be the focus of rehabilitation interventions. A patient or client could be evaluated upon admission to a program, and behaviors that are problematical could be identified and goals for treatment specified. Reevaluation at later points in the treatment would document changes in the behaviors, and, thus, progress could be assessed. Such a system can be used to evaluate patients and programs, and it is hoped that use of such a lexicon will provide a methodology for enhancing accountability.

The evaluation of the person would be conducted by interview, direct observation of the behavior, and questionnaire. During the interview, the person being evaluated would describe his behavior, what he did and what he did not do and could not do. The project directors appreciate that there is a potential measurement problem, the validity of self-report, which they have not solved yet. Who conducts the interview has not been determined and what skill level is necessary to conduct such an evaluation interview is yet to be determined. Since field testing of the lexicon is still in progress, the utility of this lexicon must be demonstrated through future research.

The Longitudinal Functional Assessment System (LFAS) (Willems 1976b) has been developed to document behavioral outcomes of rehabilitation, but it approaches the problem from an entirely different direction than does the RIP. Rather than specifying, a priori, which categories of behavior to assess, the

LFAS monitors directly whatever the person does in his everyday routine and then translates this behavior into quantitative assessments of performance.

Although still in the process of development, the LFAS is composed of seven types of data:

1. Direct observations of patient behavior while in the hospital.
2. The rest-time monitor in the hospital (developed by Halstead and described above).
3. Wheelchair odometer, both in the hospital and after discharge.
4. Telephone interview, after discharge, every ten days to obtain a behavioral diary for that day.
5. An environmental negotiability survey, after discharge, on a monthly basis; this will document the extent to which the person can actually use the physical components of his environment.
6. Morbidity—the number and kind of medical complications that curtail activity during one year after discharge.
7. Social, vocational, and educational activities.

Selection of these categories of data and this system for obtaining the data are based on ten years of developmental research. They began with the direct daily observation of patients in the hospital, followed by the completion of daily diaries after discharge (Willems 1975, 1976b). In order to reduce the cost of collecting this information, this vast amount of data was intercorrelated, and items in the current LFAS were selected because they correlate highly with many other measures of behavior. The reliability of the data collection procedures has been assessed, and acceptable levels of validity measurements have been obtained. For example, the telephone interviews once every ten days to obtain a verbal diary correlate highly with daily written diaries kept by the patients.

Alexander (1978) and associates assessed the ability of the LFAS to predict posthospital behaviors on the basis of inhospital behaviors. Nine performance measures were factor analyzed at two periods during hospitalization. The factor scores were used as independent variables in a multiple regression procedure to predict patient performance at three months after discharge and during unscheduled rehospitalization. He found that performance indicators during the first three weeks out of bed and the last three weeks prior to discharge predicted 54 percent of the variance (correlation = 0.74) in unscheduled admissions to the hospital, 50 percent of the variance (correlation = 0.71) in independent functioning three months after discharge, and 50 percent of the variance (correlation = 0.70) in rate of activities performed outside the home setting three months after discharge.

The LFAS emphasizes the natural flow of behavior as it actually happens in the person's own environment and would seem to be essentially a system of measure of behaviors. The RIP, in contrast, appears to be a system of descriptors of behaviors. Thus, each of these projects is operating at the state of the art of outcome assessment within rehabilitation, and both of these projects should be tested by the professional community. Rather than being in competition with each other, these two systems should be used side by side, since they may be able to complement each other. The RIP has attempted to define the domain of behaviors that may be relevant to any rehabilitation case and, thus, has provided a standardized terminology that can be used in all rehabilitation centers. Consequently, if this lexicon became the standard language of all rehabilitation treatment and research efforts, we would have a basis for advancing our knowledge about rehabilitation since our definition of outcomes would be standardized. The weakness of the RIP is the measurement system.

The LFAS provides a system of measurement that has demonstrated effectiveness, but it has not emphasized the means for categorizing behaviors for comparison purposes. Thus the RIP can be helpful in defining specific treatment goals in behavioral terms, and the LFAS can assess the person's actual level of performance of these tasks in and out of the hospital. The RIP defines the molecular aspect of behavior, and the LFAS assesses the natural flow of molar behaviors.

The key to the advancement of the state of the art in rehabilitation is a system for measuring outcomes and a standard language for describing these outcomes. Since the future research in rehabilitation hinges on improved systems of measurement, these two systems should be tested thoroughly.

RECOMMENDATIONS FOR FUTURE RESEARCH

Because we know so little and we need to know so much, there are seven very broad issues that need to be researched simultaneously. Each one of these issues will require a multitude of studies over many years, but no one issue can be designated as primary or secondary. They are of equal importance because of the interaction of the influences of one area on another. Some of these issues will require longitudinal study; all will require the outcomes to be specified in behavioral terms and measured according to the principles of accepted research design.

These issues need to be studied simultaneously for several reasons. Human behavior is very complex in its determinants, and any one instance of behavior represents an interaction of many variables. These are person variables, organic variables, and environment variables. The seven research issues presented here deal primarily with person and environment variables, and neither set of variables can be considered to be more important than the other.

In addition, the rehabilitation process is a system of interacting elements which itself has an effect on the behavior of the person with spinal injury (Trieschmann and Willems 1979). We need to study this system in order to determine what changes might be made that will lead to more effective delivery of services to persons with spinal injury.

Recommendations for future research include:

1. Study the cost effectiveness of the inclusion of psychosocial training within rehabilitation versus the emphasis on physical rehabilitation exclusively.

Expert opinion and data from several studies suggest that inclusion of psychosocial services within a rehabilitation program will lead to improved functioning on the part of the person with spinal injury. Improved functioning would be defined as fewer medical complications that interrupt daily activities and increased productivity. The research needs to be longitudinal in nature and should have a large sample in order to eliminate sources of bias. Cost-benefit analyses should be included, along with multiple levels of measurement of behavior. If it is shown that psychosocial techniques do lead to improved functioning, professionals will be able to plan the rehabilitation programs accordingly.

2. Develop and test measures of outcome that emphasize direct measurements of behavior.

In order for rehabilitation systems to be evaluated and for research projects to increase our knowledge, methods of defining and measuring outcome in behavioral terms need to be perfected. The Longitudinal Functional Assessment System (LFAS) and the Rehabilitation Indicators Project (RIP) should be tested for their utility, and emphasis should be given to the further development of mechanical monitoring devices to record behavior and to give feedback in training sessions.

3. Develop and test intervention strategies that increase the functional performance of persons with spinal injury in interpersonal, vocational, and community activities.

Professionals need to study methods of improving functional performance that will give the person the skills they need to find some satisfaction in life so that they have a reason to prevent medical complications and the opportunity to be a productive member of society. Included in this research effort would be, but not limited to: social skills training; assertiveness training; work skills training (other than college education); training in survival issues such as financial planning and attendant management; training in the specifics of sexual relationships (including an evaluation of penile prostheses); applications of behavioral principles to the rehabilitation process; and the role of counseling techniques.

4. Study the process of adjustment to spinal cord injury.

The impact of spinal cord injury on behavior needs to be studied along with the kinds of adaptations that occur over time. We need longitudinal research to study the stage theory of adjustment, the emotional reaction to disability (including biochemical measures), and the role of sensory deprivation in the early stages of treatment of spinal cord injury. We need to evaluate the relevance of the locus of control dimension, the role of demographic variables on adjustment, the role of behavioral variables on death rate, and the alternations in sexual function following spinal injury. With increased knowledge in these areas, we will have identified some of the problems in functioning that our intervention strategies aim to remedy.

5. Develop and test alternative service delivery mechanisms.

Since the regional spinal injury centers treat less than 15 percent of the population with spinal injury, we should explore additional service delivery mechanisms, such as transitional living centers, cooperative living centers, homebound rehabilitation programs, the case manager approach, centers for independent living, the multistage rehabilitation approach. Through such programs we should be able to reduce the cost of spinal injury to the nation.

6. Study the process of rehabilitation.

The process of rehabilitation becomes an important environmental variable in the disabled person's life. Professionals need to assess the impact of the rehabilitation system on the behavior of the disabled person and to evaluate the methods by which we can improve the functioning of the person with a disability. We need to study the planned use of behavioral principles versus the medical model in order to test the efficacy of our procedures. We need to study the effect of rehabilitation staff behavior on patient or client behavior and evaluate alternative types of training programs for staff. We need to assess the effect of direct contingencies between staff rewards and patient performance. And we need to study methods by which we can obtain changes in the behavior of rehabilitation personnel to be consistent with the findings of research. By studying all of these areas, we will be able to provide a rehabilitation environment that will facilitate patient or client performance and will reduce the overall cost of the rehabilitation process.

7. Study the role of the financial disincentives to productivity.

The current welfare legislation contains certain provisions that inadvertently penalize efforts to become financially independent or more productive. Professionals need to study the effect of the removal of these disincentives on the productivity of a large sample of persons with disabilities in order to identify methods of reducing the cost of spinal injury to the nation.

11
An Expanded View
of Rehabilitation

A person's life is like a stream flowing down a channel; the course of the stream is not straight but marked by angles and turns. Yet the water tends to flow in one general direction. There may be occasional events that have a significant impact on the flow and direction of the stream, such as a large boulder or rock that becomes lodged in the streambed. The flow of the water is not stopped, but it may be temporarily slowed as the water searches for a way around the rock. In time, a new channel will be created and the water will again move downstream. The resultant direction of the stream may be modified somewhat but usually there will be a trend, a direction that has been determined by the flow of the stream above the boulder.

The onset of spinal injury is somewhat similar to a rock or boulder becoming lodged in a streambed. There will be a disruption to the flow of life for a while, but life goes on and the person continues to evolve in ways consistent with preinjury influences. However, the impact of the spinal injury will depend on the level and completeness of the injury, the number of preinjury rewarding activities that are still possible, the person's style of coping with stress, and the environment to which the person returns, to name just a few factors. Thus, there will be a tremendous diversity of reaction to spinal injury because of the unique combination of person, organism, and environment variables which each person represents. Unfortunately, the fact that a majority of spinal injuries occur in young males has led to an overestimation of the degree of homogeneity of this group.

Adult development does not stop because of a spinal injury. Rather, the disability will be incorporated into life and adult development will continue along many of the lines established prior to the injury. Most persons with spinal injury can look forward to marriage and family responsibilities, productive efforts, involvement in the community, and some fun and rewarding leisure time activities. Thus, life goes on and rehabilitation should prepare a person to participate in these activities which are a natural part of adulthood.

However, rehabilitation as it has been practiced has fallen short of this goal. The content of rehabilitation programs has been limited by a service delivery model that focuses on giving units of treatment to the paralysis and loss of sensation. Without a doubt, bed and wheelchair mobility, grooming, bladder and bowel management, and prevention of pressure sores are necessary for participation in adult life, but they are not sufficient for successful adult functioning. The content of rehabilitation programs has been further limited by the hospital environment which is architecturally (and unrealistically) negotiable by disabled persons but which permits little independence, decision making, or practice of the variety of social skills that are essential for success in an able-bodied world. Without a doubt, the newly injured person does not know what he needs to know and therefore advice and help with some of the major decisions constituting a rehabilitation program will be necessary. But this experience will not be sufficient training for the independent decision making of an adult who must care for his own body, select a vocational program, hire and manage an attendant, arrange for transportation, manage a home and family, and survive economically.

Thus, there has been a lack of correlation between the skills taught in rehabilitation programs and the skills needed for living as an adult. The onset of a severe physical disability is not only a physical problem; consequently, a physical solution is not sufficient. Rather, the disability segregates one from the community of one's peers. One becomes isolated, different, and unable to compete in the same activities with the same ease as prior to the injury. Measures of this isolation from society include the 12 percent incidence of suicide in one study and the 46 percent incidence of deaths associated with self-neglect in other studies.

Rehabilitation is the process of learning to live with one's disability in one's own environment. If this is true, then how can rehabilitation be considered to be those activities that occur in a hospital? Rather, rehabilitation is a dynamic process evolving over a period of many years in a disabled person's life. Consequently, to be consistent with this reality, a multistage rehabilitation program should be developed which includes a rehabilitation hospital, a transitional living center, and an intensive follow-up program.

A MULTISTAGE REHABILITATION PROGRAM

A multistage rehabilitation program would add at least two additional components to the present service delivery system. Acute medical management of spinal injury would occur within the traditional rehabilitation center as would physical rehabilitation. However, a transitional living experience and follow-up in the community would provide an opportunity to practice ADL and mobility skills and to learn psychosocial survival skills.

The Traditional Rehabilitation Center

The traditional rehabilitation center would be only the first step in a rehabilitation program. The emphasis here would be on medical management of the injury and the teaching of ADL and mobility skills, but some changes within the rehabilitation center would be desirable. Even though rehabilitation hospitals must coordinate the activities of a large number of personnel, which leads to schedules and artificial divisions of labor, there are many ways in which the disabled person can play a more decisive role in the rehabilitation program. The key to these changes is the behavior of many rehabilitation personnel toward the disabled person. Although most personnel have a good and often warm relationship with a disabled person on a one-to-one basis, these professionals have certain ways of behaving toward the population of disabled persons that are extremely impersonal and, unintentionally, demeaning.

Language is one indication of attitudes toward people. Customarily, we refer to the "para in bed 4" or the "quad on the tilt-table" rather than to John Smith, who has a paraplegia, or Mary Jones, who has a quadriplegia. In general, we talk of paras and quads rather than of *persons* with paraplegia and *persons* with quadriplegia which takes just a little bit longer to say. Professionals often will continue to refer to disabled persons as "patients" despite the fact that these persons are not hospitalized. Thus, it appears that to some professionals, once a patient, always a patient, and the disabled person is never allowed to graduate to personhood. Many professionals who expect to be called "Doctor," often call a disabled person by his or her first name. This occurs less frequently among professionals without the doctor title, yet this discrepancy in mode of address occurs often enough to be a concern. When the team gives information to the disabled person and his or her family, very frequently team members will talk to the family *about* the person rather than talk *to* the person in the presence of the family. Such statements as, "he is doing better in transfers," or "she is now independent in bed mobility," rather than, "you are doing much better in transfers" or "you are now independent in bed mobility" exemplify this problem.

These situations can be observed daily in every rehabilitation center around the country. Collectively, these ways of talking to and about persons with disabilities send a message to the disabled person that he or she is less worthy of respect since the injury. That is not the intention, but that is the effect at a time when the injured person is fearing that he is less worthy than he used to be.

Other behaviors of hospital personnel can add to the person's feeling that he or she is worthy of less respect since the disability. In teaching hospitals there is always the problem of how to transmit information from the teacher to student. Demonstration of techniques on a hospitalized patient is a necessary part of the teaching process; however, how this is introduced and implemented can influence the impact on the hospitalized person's sense of respect. Morning rounds on the ward can be the occasion for teaching. However, some professionals will interrupt a patient's breakfast by pulling the tray away without asking permission, conduct part of a physical exam, and walk away leaving the breakfast tray out of reach. During many types of rounds, the professionals may talk *about* the disabled person in his or her presence without more than a casual "hello." The person is not the beneficiary of the discussion nor included in it but only the subject of the discussion. All of these teaching activities could be conducted in the context of basic courtesy and old-fashioned good manners and have even more value as a training device. Students model the behavior of their professors and the modeling of bad manners occurs only too often.

Thus, procedures in traditional rehabilitation centers should be modified to show more respect for the person with the disability. The person with the disability should be included in the team conferences so he can hear the progress reports and participate in the decisions. At one very fine hospital, a progress conference is held every two weeks, and the disabled person and family are expected to participate. Inclusion of the disabled person and family *does not* lengthen the conference time because information is exchanged efficiently and frequently.

The focus of the efforts at the traditional rehabilitation center would be ADL and mobility training, but these techniques would be taught using a learning model of service delivery. Because it was recognized that the ability to get on and off a toilet was not sufficient for successful adult life, further training at a transitional living center, stage two, would be recommended.

The Transitional Living Center

Discharge from the traditional rehabilitation center occurs at that point when the disabled person can do as much of his or her ADL and mobility as seems feasible at the time. However, the correlation between *can do* and *does do* is often not high. After a severe physical disability, it may take a year or two for all of these new procedures to become a fairly automatic part of life. In addition, there are other skills that need to be learned, such as putting able-bodied persons at ease, negotiating the community despite architectural barriers, hiring and managing an attendant, financial planning, job seeking, etc.

The focus of a transitional living center is the *application* of the ADL and mobility to everyday life and the learning of the skills that are necessary for interpersonal success as an adult. The timing of this phase of rehabilitation will depend upon the individual, some needing and desiring such experience immediately after discharge from the rehabilitation center and some needing time at home first. In either case, this phase should be a mandatory part of all rehabilitation programs. This concept has been successfully demonstrated using a residential facility, but lack of such a facility need not interfere with the learning of many of these interpersonal skills.

Follow-up in the Community

Following these two somewhat formalized phases of rehabilitation, the best learning occurs in one's own community. As with all educational programs, the graduate discovers that he or she has only been given the techniques to solve life's problems but not the solutions to the problems themselves. The addition of a transitional living center phase to rehabilitation does not guarantee success. But it does provide the disabled person with additional skills to use in living with the disability. However, there will be fluctuations in the person's degree of success at coping with life, similar to the experiences of able-bodied persons. Thus, a system of follow-up services focusing on problem prevention rather than crisis intervention is needed. Such services should emphasize the utilization of community resources to assist the disabled person rather than the development of new services for the disabled population alone.

The use of telephone interviews and environmental negotiability surveys, as described in chapter 10, could be very helpful as a means of detecting difficulties before they become major problems. Nevertheless, a balance must be maintained between solutions provided by professionals in times of crisis and solutions achieved by disabled persons to prevent crisis. Independence in problem solving is one of the ultimate criteria of rehabilitation success. This balance will be maintained if the professional truly respects the disabled person and if procedures have been established for consumer involvement.

The multistage rehabilitation concept is based on the recognition that successful adult functioning following the onset of a severe disability requires more than ADL and mobility techniques. The psychosocial impact of a disability is tremendous and specific attention must be given to these issues. Therefore, the need for psychologists to be intimately involved in all phases of the rehabilitation process is greater than ever before.

THE ROLE OF THE PSYCHOLOGIST IN TREATMENT OF SPINAL INJURY

The role of the psychologist in the treatment of spinal injury has evolved over many years as the emphasis in rehabilitation has shifted from survival of the disabled person to psychosocial integration into the community. As has been documented in this book, persons with spinal injury do not have psychological problems per se but rather they have tremendous reality problems as they learn to live with a disability. Rehabilitation is a learning process in which the individual's personal strengths and assets are developed and used to work around the liabilities imposed by the physical paralysis. Within this context, then, the psychologist's skills are essential to the rehabilitation team's efforts. Thus, the psychologist contributes to the rehabilitation process in at least four ways (Trieschmann 1978):

1. Consultation with the rehabilitation team.
   a. Application of the principles of learning to the rehabilitation process.
   b. Identification of important psychosocial issues in individual cases.
2. Research into the rehabilitation process.
3. Psychological evaluation of the disabled person's strengths and assets.
4. Designing and implementing intervention strategies to utilize the person's strengths and assets.

In order to reduce the incidence of deaths from self-destructive actions in the spinal injury population, there must be increased emphasis on the psychosocial issues of disability. Thus, the psychologist and others trained in the behavioral disciplines must become an increasingly visible part of rehabilitation programs. Our knowledge about the process of adjustment to spinal injury is imperfect. Nevertheless, if we forget the myths about disability and truly listen to the person with a disability, we can learn and work together to help the person go through his very normal reaction to an abnormal situation.

Bibliography

Abramson, A.; Kutner, B.; Rosenberg, P.; Berger, R.; and Weiner, H. A therapeutic community in a general hospital: Adaptation to a rehabilitation service. *Journal of Chronic Diseases,* 1963, **16,** 179-86.

Albrecht, G., and Higgins, P. Rehabilitation success: The interrelationships of multiple criteria. *Journal of Health and Social Behavior,* 1977, **18,** 36-45.

Alexander, J. Performance assessment system in spinal cord injury. Unpublished doctoral dissertation, University of Houston, 1978.

Anderson, T. Educational frame of reference: An additional model for rehabilitation medicine. *Archives of Physical Medicine and Rehabilitation,* 1978, **59,** 203-6.

Anderson, T., and Andberg, M. Psychosocial factors associated with incidence of pressure sores on spinal cord injured patients. Paper presented at American Congress of Rehabilitation Medicine, Miami Beach, October 1977.

Anderson, T., and Cole, T. Sexual counseling of the physically disabled. *Postgraduate Medicine,* 1975, **58,** 117-25.

Anthony, W. Societal rehabilitation: Changing society's attitudes toward the physically and mentally disabled. *Rehabilitation Psychology,* 1972, **19,** 117-26.

Antler, L.; Lee, M.: Zaretsky, H.; Pezenik, D.; and Halberstam, J. Attitudes of rehabilitation patients towards the wheelchair. *Journal of Psychology,* 1969, **73,** 45-52.

Arnhoff, F., and Mehl, M. Body image deterioration in paraplegia. *Journal of Nervous and Mental Diseases,* 1963, **137,** 88-92.

Athelstan, G., and Crewe, N. Patterns of adjustment to severe physical disability. *Archives of Physical Medicine and Rehabilitation,* 1977, **58,** 533, abstract.

Athelstan, G., and Crewe, N. Psychological adjustment to spinal cord injury as related to manner of onset of disability. *Rehabilitation Counseling Bulletin,* in press.

Averill, J. Personal control over aversive stimuli and its relationship to stress. *Psychological Bulletin,* 1973, **80,** 286-303.

Bandura, A. *Principles of behavior modification.* New York: Holt, Rinehart, and Winston, 1969.

Barber, T. *Pitfalls in human research.* New York: Pergamon Press, 1976.

Barker, R. *Ecological psychology.* Stanford, Calif.: Stanford University Press, 1968.

Barker, R. On the nature of the environment. In H. Proshansky, W. Ittelson, and L. Rivlin (Eds.), *Environmental psychology: People and their physical settings.* New York: Holt, Rinehart, and Winston, 1976.

Barrie, D. Non-medical management of spinal cord injury. *International Journal of Paraplegia,* 1973, **11,** 96-98.

Bass, R. Group counseling in vocational adjustment. *Journal of Rehabilitation,* 1969, **35,** 25-28.

Becker, M.; Abrams, K.; and Onder, J. Goal setting: A joint patient-staff method. *Archives of Physical Medicine and Rehabilitation,* 1974, **55,** 87-89.

Bell, A. Attitudes toward nudity by social class. *Medical Aspects of Human Sexuality,* 1969, **3,** 101-10.

Berger, S., and Garrett, J. Psychological problems of the paraplegic patient. *Journal of Rehabilitation,* 1952, **18,** 15-17.

Berk, S., and Feibel, J. The unmet psychosocial and family needs of stroke survivors. Paper presented at the American Congress of Rehabilitation Medicine, New Orleans, November 1978.

Berkman, A.; Weissman, R.; and Frielich, M. Sexual adjustment of spinal cord injured veterans living in the community. *Archives of Physical Medicine and Rehabilitation*, 1978, **59**, 29-33.

Berni, R., and Fordyce, W. *Behavior modification and the nursing process*. St. Louis: C. V. Mosby Co., 1973.

Berscheid, E., and Walster, E. Physical attractiveness. *Advances in Experimental Social Psychology*, 1974, **7**, 157-215.

Bors, E. Phantom limbs of patients with spinal cord injury. *Archives of Neurology and Psychiatry*, 1951, **66**, 610-31.

Bourestom, N., and Howard, M. Personality characteristics of three disability groups. *Archives of Physical Medicine and Rehabilitation*, 1965, **46**, 626-32.

Braakman, R.; Orbaan, J.; and Dishoeck, M. Information in the early stages after spinal cord injury. *International Journal of Paraplegia*, 1976, **14**, 95-100.

Bregman, S., and Hadley, R. Sexual adjustment and feminine attractiveness among spinal cord injured women. *Archives of Physical Medicine and Rehabilitation*, 1976, **57**, 448-50.

Brockway, J. MMPI correlates of medical complications in spinal cord injury. Paper presented at American Congress of Rehabilitation Medicine, New Orleans, November 1978.

Brockway, J., and Steger, J. Sexual attitude and information questionnaire: Reliability and validity in a spinal cord injured population. Paper presented at American Congress of Rehabilitation Medicine, New Orleans, November 1978.

Brown, B., and Chanin, I. *Patterns of education and employment: Rehabilitants from severe spinal cord injury, FY 1972-73*. Rehabilitation Research Reports, no. 30, Department of Rehabilitation, Sacramento, Calif., June 1, 1974.

Buck, F. The influence of parental disability on children: an exploratory investigation of the adult children of spinal cord injured fathers. Doctoral Dissertation, University of Arizona, 1980.

Bunney, W.; Mason, J.; and Hamburg, D. Correlation between behavioral variables and urinary 17-Hydroxy-corticosteroids in depressed patients. *Psychosomatic Medicine*, 1965, **27**, 299-308.

Burke, D. Pain in paraplegia. *International Journal of Paraplegia*, 1973, **10**, 297-313.

Carlson, C. Cognitive structure, goal characteristics, and life satisfaction following spinal cord injury. Doctoral dissertation, University of Colorado, 1974.

Carlson, R. *The end of medicine*. New York: John Wiley and Sons, 1975.

Carmack, B. Personal communication, January 10, 1977.

Carter, R. Personal communication, July 7, 1977.

Caywood, T. A quadriplegic young man looks at treatment. *Journal of Rehabilitation*, 1974, **49**, 22-25.

Chanin, I., and Brown, B. *Incidence of disability and characteristics of clients closed from plan with severe spinal cord injury, FY 1972-73*. Rehabilitation Research Reports, no. 34, Department of Rehabilitation, Sacramento, Calif., December 30, 1975.

Christophersen, V. Role modifications of the disabled male. *American Journal of Nursing*, 1968, **68**, 290-93.

Cimperman, A., and Dunn, M. Group therapy with spinal cord injured patients: A case study. *Rehabilitation Psychology*, 1974, **21**, 44-48.

Clore, G., and Jeffrey, K. Emotional role playing, attitude change, and attraction toward a disabled person. *Journal of Personality and Social Psychology*, 1972, **23**, 105-11.

Cobb, S. Social support as a moderator of life stress. *Psychosomatic Medicine*, 1976, **38**, 300-314.

Cogswell, B. Rehabilitation of the paraplegic: Processes of socialization. *Sociological Inquiry*, 1967, **37**, 11-26.

Cogswell, B. Self socialization: Readjustment of paraplegics in the community. *Journal of Rehabilitation,* 1968, **34,** 11-13, 35.

Cole, T. Sexuality and physical disabilities. *Archives of Sexual Behavior,* 1975, **4,** 389-403.

Cole, T.; Chilgren, R.; and Rosenberg, P. A new programme of sex education and counseling for spinal cord injured adults and health care professionals. *International Journal of Paraplegia,* 1973, **11,** 111-24.

Cole, T., and Stevens, M. Rehabilitation professionals and sexual counseling for spinal cord injured adults. *Archives of Sexual Behavior,* 1975, **4,** 631-38.

Comarr, E. Marriage and divorce among patients with spinal cord injury, I. *Journal of the Indian Medical Profession,* 1962, **9,** 4353-59.

Comarr, E. Marriage and divorce among patients with spinal cord injury, II-V. *Journal of the Indian Medical Profession,* 1963, **9,** 4162-68, 4181-86, 4378-84, 4424-30.

Comarr, A., and Vigue, M. Sexual counseling among male and female patients with spinal cord and/or cauda equina injury, Part I. *American Journal of Physical Medicine,* 1978a, **57,** 107-22.

Comarr, A., and Vigue, M. Sexual counseling among male and female patients with spinal cord and/or cauda equina injury, Part II. *American Journal of Physical Medicine,* 1978b, **57,** 215-27.

Comprehensive service needs study. Urban Institute, Washington, D.C., June 23, 1975.

Comprehensive service needs study: Executive summary. Urban Institute, Washington, D. C., June 23, 1975.

Conomy, J. Disorders of body image after spinal cord injury. *Neurology,* 1973, **23,** 842-50.

Consumer conference on research issues in the psychological, social, and vocational adjustment to spinal cord injury. Easter Seal Society of Los Angeles County, Los Angeles, June 11, 1977.

Cook, D. Psychological aspects of spinal cord injury. *Rehabilitation Counseling Bulletin,* 1976, **19,** 535-43.

Costello, C. Depression: Loss of reinforcers or loss of reinforcer effectiveness? *Behavior Therapy,* 1972, **3,** 240-47.

Crase, C. Major competitive sports for wheelchair athletes. *Rehabilitation Record,* 1972, **13,** 26-29.

Crewe, N.; Athelstan, G.; and Bower, A. *Employment after spinal cord injury: A handbook for counselors.* Minneapolis: Department of Physical Medicine and Rehabilitation, University of Minnesota, 1978.

Crewe, N.; Athelstan, G.; and Krumberger, J. Marriages after spinal cord injury. Paper presented at American Congress of Rehabilitation Medicine, New Orleans, November 1978.

Crewe, N.; Athelstan, G.; and Meadows, G. Vocational diagnosis through assessment of functional limitations. *Archives of Physical Medicine and Rehabilitation,* 1975, **56,** 513-16.

Crigler, L. Sexual concerns of the spinal cord injured. *Nursing Clinician in North America,* 1974, **9,** 703-16.

Cull, J., and Hardy, R. *Behavior modification in rehabilitation settings.* Springfield, Ill.: Charles C. Thomas, 1974.

Cull, J., and Hardy, R. *Physical medicine and rehabilitation approaches in spinal cord injury.* Springfield, Ill.: Charles C. Thomas, 1977.

Cull, J., and Smith, O. A preliminary note on demographic and personality correlates of decubitus ulcer incidence. *Journal of Psychology,* 1973, **85,** 225-27.

Das, S. Some psychological problems of quadriplegics. *Medical Journal of Australia,* 1969, **2,** 562-64.

Davis, F. Deviance disavowal: The management of strained interaction by the visibly handicapped. *Social Problems,* 1961, **9,** 120-32.

Dembo, T.; Leviton, G.; and Wright, B. Adjustment to misfortune—A problem of social-psychological rehabilitation. *Rehabilitation Psychology,* 1975, **22,** 1-100.

Deyoe, F. Marriage and family patterns with long-term spinal cord injury. *International Journal of Paraplegia,* 1972a, **10,** 219-24.

Deyoe, F. Spinal cord injury: Long-term follow-up of veterans. *Archives of Physical Medicine and Rehabilitation,* 1972b, **53,** 523-29.

Diamond, M.; Weiss, A.; and Grynbaum, B. The unmotivated patient. *Archives of Physical Medicine and Rehabilitation,* 1968, **49,** 281-84.

Diller, L.; Fordyce, W.; Jacobs, D.; and Brown, M. Rehabilitation indicators: A method for enhancing accountability and the provision of rehabilitation services. Project Summary, New York University Medical Center, 1977.

Dimond, R., and Hirt, M. Body involvement among schizophrenics, normals, and paraplegics. *Social Behavior and Personality,* 1973, **1,** 33-34.

Dinardo, Q. Psychological adjustment to spinal cord injury. Doctoral dissertation, University of Houston, 1971.

Dinsdale, S.; Lesser, A.; and Judd, F. Critical psychosocial variables affecting outcome in a regional spinal cord centre. *Proceedings of the Eighteenth Veterans Administration Spinal Cord Injury Conference,* 1971, **18,** 193-96.

Doob, A., and Ecker, B. Stigma and compliance. *Journal of Personality and Social Psychology,* 1970, **14,** 302-4.

Dunn, D. Adjustment to spinal cord injury in the rehabilitation hospital setting. Doctoral dissertation, University of Maryland, 1969.

Dunn, M. Social discomfort in the patient with spinal cord injury. *Archives of Physical Medicine and Rehabilitation,* 1977, **58,** 257-60.

Dunn, M., and Davis, R. The perceived effects of marijuana on spinal cord injured males. *International Journal of Paraplegia,* 1974, **12,** 175.

Dunn, M.; Van Horn, E.; and Herman, S. A comparison of three training procedures for spinal cord injury social skills. Paper presented at American Congress of Rehabilitation Medicine, Miami Beach, November 1977.

Dvonch, P.; Kaplan, L.; Grynbaum, B.; and Rusk, H. Vocational findings in post disability employment of patients with spinal cord dysfunction. *Archives of Physical Medicine and Rehabilitation,* 1965, **46,** 761-66.

Edelstein, B., and Eisler, R. Effects of modeling and modeling with instructions and feedback on the behavioral components of social skills. *Behavior Therapy,* 1976, **7,** 382-89.

Eisenberg, M., and Rustad, L. Sex education and counseling program on a spinal cord injury service. *Archives of Physical Medicine and Rehabilitation,* 1976, **57,** 135-40.

El Ghatit, A., and Hanson, R. Outcome of marriages existing at the time of a male's spinal cord injury. *Journal of Chronic Disease,* 1975, **28,** 383-88.

El Ghatit, A., and Hanson, R. Marriage and divorce after spinal cord injury. *Archives of Physical Medicine and Rehabilitation,* 1976, **57,** 470-72.

El Ghatit, A., and Hanson, R. Variables associated with obtaining and sustaining employment among spinal cord injured males: A follow-up of 760 veterans. *Journal of Chronic Disease,* 1978, **31,** 363-69.

English, R. Correlates of stigma towards physically disabled persons. *Rehabilitation Research and Practice Review,* 1971, **2,** 1-17.

Euse, F. An application of covert positive reinforcement for modification of attitudes toward physically disabled persons. Doctoral dissertation, Auburn University, 1975.

Evans, J. On disturbance of the body image in paraplegia. *Brain,* 1962, **85,** 687-700.

Evans, R.; Halar, E.; DeFreece, A.; and Larsen, G. Multi-disciplinary approach to sex education of spinal cord injured patients. *Physical Therapy,* 1976, **56,** 541-45.

Felton, J. Blocks to employment of paralytics. *Rehabilitation Record,* 1964, **5,** 35-37.

Felton, J., and Litman, M. Study of employment of 222 men with spinal cord injury. *Archives of Physical Medicine and Rehabilitation,* 1965, **46,** 809-14.

Ferdinand, T. Sex behavior and the American class structure: A mosaic. *Medical Aspects of Human Sexuality,* 1969, **3,** 34-46.

Fink, S.; Skipper, J.; and Hallenback, P. Physical disability and problems in marriage. *Journal of Marriage and the Family*, 1968, **30**, 64-74.

Fitting, M.; Salisbury, S.; Davies, N.; and Mayclin, D. Self concept and sexuality of spinal cord injured women. *Archives of Sexual Behavior*, 1978, **7**, 143-56.

Flynn, R., and Salomone, P. Performance of the MMPI in predicting rehabilitation outcome: A discriminant analysis, double cross-validation assessment. *Rehabilitation Literature*, 1977, **38**, 12-14, 15.

Ford, C., and Beach, F. *Patterns of sexual behavior*. New York: Harper and Brothers and Paul B. Hoeber, Medical Books, 1951.

Fordyce, W. Personality characteristics of men with spinal cord injury as related to manner of onset of disability. *Archives of Physical Medicine and Rehabilitation*, 1964, **45**, 321-25.

Fordyce, W. Behavioral methods in rehabilitation. In W. Neff (Ed.), *Rehabilitation Psychology*. Washington, D.C. : American Psychological Association, 1971.

Fordyce, W. Research on influencing level of patient participation in the rehabilitation process. *Selected research topics in spinal cord injury rehabilitation*. Grant no. 16-P-56813/6-13, Houston, Texas: Texas Institute for Rehabilitation and Research, 1975.

Fordyce, W. *Behavioral methods for chronic pain and illness*. St. Louis: C. V. Mosby Co., 1976.

Fordyce, W.; Fowler, R.; Lehmann, J.; DeLateur, B.; Sand, P.; and Trieschmann, R. Treatment of chronic pain by operant conditioning. *Archives of Physical Medicine and Rehabilitation*, 1973, **54**, 399-408.

Fordyce, W.; Fowler, R.; Sand, P.; and Trieschmann, R. Behavioral systems analyzed. *Journal of Rehabilitation*, 1971, **37**, 29-34.

Frank, J. *Persuasion and healing: A comparative study of psychotherapy*. New York: Schocken Books, 1974.

Franklin, B., and Osborne, H. *Research methods: Issues and insights*. Belmont, Calif.: Wadsworth Publishing Co, 1971.

French, D.; McDowell, R.; and Keith, R. Participant observation as a patient in a rehabilitation hospital. *Rehabilitation Psychology*, 1972, **19**, 89-95.

Frieden, L., and Halstead, L. Application of unobtrusive longitudinal monitoring techniques to assess gross behavioral activity in a noninstitutional setting. Paper presented at American Congress of Rehabilitation Medicine, San Diego, November 1976.

Friedson, E. Disability as social deviance. In M. Sussman (Ed.), *Sociology and rehabilitation*. Washington, D. C.: American Sociological Association, 1965.

Friedson, E. *Profession of medicine: A study of the sociology of applied knowledge*. New York: Harper and Row, 1970.

Garrett, J. Professionalism in rehabilitation in the 1980's. *Archives of Physical Medicine and Rehabilitation*, 1976, **57**, 93-97.

Geis, G. A therapeutic aquatics program for quadriplegic patients. *American Corrective Therapy Journal*, 1975, **29**, 155-57.

Geisler, W.; Jousse, A.; and Wynne-Jones, M. Vocational re-establishment of patients with spinal cord injury. *Medical Services Journal of Canada*, 1966a, **22**, 698-710.

Geisler, W.; Jousse, A.; and Wynne-Jones, M. Vocational re-establishment of patients with spinal cord injury. *Prosthetics International*, 1966b, **2**, 29-38.

Goffman, Erving. *Asylums*. Garden City, N.Y.: Anchor Books, Doubleday, 1961.

Goffman, Erving. *Stigma*. Englewood Cliffs, N.J.: Prentice-Hall, 1963.

Goldberg, R., and Freed, M. Vocational adjustment, interests, work values, and career plans of persons with spinal cord injuries. *Scandinavian Journal of Rehabilitation Medicine*, 1973, **5**, 3-11.

Goldberg, R., and Freed, M. The vocational development, interests, values, adjustment, and rehabilitation outlook of spinal cord patients: A four-year follow-up. Paper presented at American Congress of Rehabilitation Medicine, San Diego, November 1976.

Goldiamond, I. A diary of self-modification. *Psychology Today,* November 1973, **7**, 95-102.

Goldiamond, I. Coping and adaptive behaviors of the disabled. In G. Albrecht (Ed.), *The sociology of physical disability and rehabilitation.* Pittsburgh: University of Pittsburgh Press, 1976.

Goldstein, A. *Structured learning therapy: Toward a psychotherapy for the poor.* New York: Academic Press, 1973.

Golightly-Eberly, C. Personal communication, February 17, 1978.

Golightly, C., and Reinehr, R. Fantasy production of quadriplegic males: A preliminary investigation. *American Corrective Therapy Journal,* 1972, **26**, 47-49.

Griffith, E.; Timms, R.; and Tomko, M. *Sexual problems of patients with spinal injuries: An annotated bibliography.* Department of Physical Medicine and Rehabilitation, University of Cincinnati, Cincinnati, Ohio, March 1972.

Griffith, E.; Tomko, M.; and Timms, R. Sexual function in spinal cord injured patients: A review. *Archives of Physical Medicine and Rehabilitation,* 1973, **54**, 539-43.

Griffith, E., and Trieschmann, R. Sexual function in females with spinal cord injury. *Archives of Physical Medicine and Rehabilitation,* 1975, **56**, 18-21.

Griffith, E., and Trieschmann, R. Sexual functioning in patients with physical disorders. In J. Meyer (Ed.), *Clinical management of sexual disorders.* Baltimore: Williams and Wilkins, 1976.

Griffith, E., and Trieschmann, R. Sexual function restoration in the physically disabled: Use of a private hospital room. *Archives of Physical Medicine and Rehabilitation,* 1977, **58**, 368-69.

Griffith, E., and Trieschmann, R. Use of a private hospital room in restoring sexual function to the physically disabled. *Sexuality and Disability,* 1978, **1**, 179-83.

Griffith, E.; Trieschmann, R.; Hohmann, G.; Cole, T.; Tobis, J.; and Cummings, V. Sexual dysfunctions associated with physical disabilities. *Archives of Physical Medicine and Rehabilitation,* 1975, **56**, 8-13.

Grynbaum, B.; Kaplan, L.; Lloyd, K.; and Rusk, H. Methodology and initial findings in a follow-up study of spinal cord dysfunction. *Archives of Physical Medicine and Rehabilitation,* 1963, **44**, 208-15.

Gunther, M. Emotional aspects. In R. Reuge (Ed.), *Spinal cord injuries.* Springfield, Ill.: Charles C. Thomas, 1969.

Guttmann, L. Significance of sport in rehabilitation of spinal paraplegics and tetraplegics. *Journal of the American Medical Association,* 1976, **236**, 195-97.

Guttmann, L., and Mehra, N. Experimental studies on the value of archery in paraplegics. *International Journal of Paraplegia,* 1973, **11**, 159-65.

Hallin, R. Follow-up of paraplegics and tetraplegics after comprehensive rehabilitation. *International Journal of Paraplegia,* 1968, **6**, 128-34.

Halstead, L. Wheelchair odometer: A method for quantitating patients' mobility in wheelchairs. *Archives of Physical Medicine and Rehabilitation,* 1973, **54**, 39-42.

Halstead, L. Longitudinal unobtrusive measurements in rehabilitation. *Archives of Physical Medicine and Rehabilitation,* 1976, **54**, 189-93.

Halstead, L.; Halstead, M.; Salhoot, J.; Stock, D.; and Sparks, R. An interdisciplinary program on human sexuality for health care professionals and the physically handicapped. *Southern Medical Journal,* 1976, **69**, 1352-55.

Halstead, L.; Halstead, M.; Salhoot, J.; Stock, D.; and Sparks, R. A hospital based program in human sexuality. *Archives of Physical Medicine and Rehabilitation,* 1977, **58**, 409-12.

Halstead, L.; Halstead, M.; Salhoot, J.; Stock, D.; and Sparks, R. Sexual attitudes, behavior, and satisfaction for able bodied and disabled participants attending workshops in human sexuality. *Archives of Physical Medicine and Rehabilitation,* 1978, **59**, 497-501.

Handicapped persons pilot project: Residential care needs. California State Department of Public Health, Bureau of Chronic Diseases, January 1969.

Hanson, R., and Franklin, M. Sexual loss in relation to other functional losses for spinal cord injured males. *Archives of Physical Medicine and Rehabilitation,* 1976, **57**, 291-303.

Harlow, H. *Learning to Love*. New York: Ballantine Books, 1971.

Harris, P.; Patel, S.; Greer, W.; and Naughton, J. Psychological and social reactions to acute spinal paralysis. *International Journal of Paraplegia*, 1973, **11**, 132-36.

Heijn, C. Some emotional factors influencing rehabilitation in patients with spinal cord injury. *Proceedings of the 18th Veterans Administration Spinal Cord Conference*, 1971, **18**, 196-98.

Heijn, C., and Granger, G. Understanding motivational patterns—Early identification aids rehabilitation. *Journal of Rehabilitation*, 1974, **40**, 26-28.

Heilporn, A., and Noel, G. Reflections on the consciousness of disability and somatognosis in cases of acute spinal injuries. *International Journal of Paraplegia*, 1968, **6**, 122-27.

Held, J.; Cole, T.; Held, C.; Anderson, C.; and Chilgren, R. Sexual attitude reassessment workshops: Effect on spinal cord injured adults, their partners, and rehabilitation professionals. *Archives of Physical Medicine and Rehabilitation*, 1975, **56**, 14-18.

Hersen, M., and Bellack, A. A multiple-baseline analysis of social skills training in chronic schizophrenics. *Journal of Applied Behavior Analysis*, 1976, **9**, 239-45.

Hirschenfang, S., and Benton, J. Rorschach responses of paraplegic and quadriplegic patients. *International Journal of Paraplegia*, 1966, **4**, 40-42.

Hohmann, G. Some effects of spinal cord lesions on experienced emotional feelings. *Psychophysiology*, 1966, **3**, 143-56.

Hohmann, G. Considerations in management of psychosexual readjustment in the cord injured male. *Rehabilitation Psychology*, 1972, **19**, 50-58.

Hohmann, G. Psychological aspects of treatment and rehabilitation of the spinal injured person. *Clinical Orthopedics*, 1975, **112**, 81-88.

Hohmann, G. Personal communication, November 1, 1977.

Hohmann, G. Personal communication, January 6, 1978a.

Hohmann, G. Personal communication, April 4, 1978b.

Hopkins, M. Patterns of self-destruction among the orthopedically disabled. *Rehabilitation Research and Practice Review*, 1971, **3,** 5-16.

Howard J., and Strauss, A. (Eds.) *Humanizing health care*. New York: John Wiley and Sons, 1975.

Illich, I. *Medical nemesis: The expropriation of health*. New York: Pantheon Books, 1976.

Ince, L. *Behavior modification in rehabilitation medicine*. Springfield, Ill.; Charles C. Thomas, 1976.

Jasnos, T., and Hakmiller, K. Some effects of lesion level and emotional cues on affective expression in spinal cord patients. *Psychological Reports*, 1975, **37**, 859-70.

Jochheim, K., and Strohkindl, H. The value of particular sports for the wheelchair disabled in maintaining health of the paraplegic. *International Journal of Paraplegia*, 1973, **11**, 173-98.

Johnson, E.; Roberts, C.; and Godwin, H. Self-medication for a rehabilitation ward. *Archives of Physical Medicine and Rehabilitation*, 1970, **51**, 300-303.

Jones, R., and Sisk, D. Early perceptions of orthopedic disability: A developmental study. *Rehabilitation Literature*, 1970, **31**, 34-38.

Kahn, E. Social functioning of the patient with spinal cord injury. *Physical Therapy*, 1969, **49**, 757-62.

Kalb, M. An examination of the relationship between hospital ward behaviors and post-discharge behaviors in the spinal cord injury patients. Doctoral dissertation, University of Houston, 1971.

Kanfer, F., and Goldstein, A. *Helping people change*. New York: Pergamon Press, 1975.

Kanfer, F., and Karoly, P. Self-control: A behavioristic excursion into the lion's den. *Annual Review of Behavior Therapy*, 1973, **1,** 396-415.

Kaplan, L.; Powell, B.; Grynbaum, B.; and Rusk, H. (Eds.) *Comprehensive follow-up study of spinal cord dysfunction and its resultant disabilities*. New York University Medical Center, Institute of Rehabilitation Medicine, New York, 1966.

Karan, O., and Gardner, W. Vocational rehabilitation practices: A behavioral analysis. *Rehabilitation Literature*, 1973, **34**, 290-98.

Katz, R., and Zlutnick, S. *Behavior therapy and health care*. New York: Pergamon Press, 1975.

Keith, R. A. The need for a new model in rehabilitation. *Journal of Chronic Disease*, 1968, **21**, 281-86.

Keith, R. A. Physical rehabilitation: Is it ready for the revolution? *Rehabilitation Literature*, 1969, **30**, 170-73.

Keith, R. A. The comprehensive rehabilitation center as a rehabilitation model. *Inquiry*, 1971, **8** (3).

Keith, R. A. The effect of social control on rehabilitation treatment. Paper presented at the American Sociological Association, New Orleans, August 1972.

Kemp, B., and Vash, C. Productivity after injury in a sample of spinal cord injured persons: A pilot study. *Journal of Chronic Disease*, 1971, **24**, 259-75.

Kendall, P.; Edinger, J.; and Eberly, C. Taylor's MMPI correction factor for spinal cord injury: Empirical endorsement. *Journal of Consulting and Clinical Psychology*, 1978, **46**, 370-71.

Kerr, N. Staff expectations for disabled persons: Helpful or harmful. *Rehabilitation Counseling Bulletin*, 1970, **14**, 85-94.

Kerr, W., and Thompson, M. Acceptance of disability of sudden onset in paraplegia. *International Journal of Paraplegia*, 1972, **10**, 94-102.

Kinsey, A.; Poneroy, W.; and Martin, C. *Sexual behavior in the human male*. Philadelphia: W. B. Saunders, 1948.

Kiresuk, T. Goal attainment scaling at a county mental health service. *Evaluation*, 1973, special monograph, no. 1.

Kiresuk, T., and Sherman, R. Goal attainment scaling: A general method for evaluating comprehensive community mental health programs. *Community Mental Health Journal*, 1968, **4**, 443-53.

Klas, L. A study of the relationship between depression and factors in the rehabilitation process of the hospitalized spinal cord injured patient. Doctoral dissertation, University of Utah, 1970.

Kleck, R. Emotional arousal in interactions with stigmatized persons. *Psychological Reports*, 1966, **19**, 1226.

Kleck, R. Physical stigma and nonverbal cues emitted in face-to-face interaction. *Human Relations*, 1968, **21**, 19-28.

Kleck, R. Physical stigma and task oriented interactions. *Human Relations*, 1969, **22**, 53-60.

Kleck, R.; Ono, H.; and Hastorf, A. The effects of physical deviance upon face-to-face interaction. *Human Relations*, 1966, **19**, 425-36.

Klein, R.; Dean, A.; and Bogdonoff, M. The impact of illness upon the spouse. *Journal of Chronic Disease*, 1967, **20**, 241-48.

Knorr, N., and Bull, J. Spinal cord injury: Psychiatric considerations. *Maryland State Medical Journal*, 1970, **19**, 105-8.

Kolb, L. *Modern clinical psychiatry*. 8th ed. Philadelphia: W.B. Saunders, 1973.

Kunce, J., and Worley, B. Interest patterns, accidents, and disability. *Journal of Clinical Psychology*, 1966, **22**, 105-7.

Kutner, B. Milieu therapy in rehabilitation medicine. *Journal of Rehabilitation*, 1968, **34**, 14-17.

Kutner, B. Professional anti-therapy. *Journal of Rehabilitation*, 1969, **35**, 16-18.

Kutner, B. The social psychology of disability. In W. Neff (Ed.), *Rehabilitation Psychology*. Washington, D. C.: American Psychological Association, 1971a.

Kutner, B. Rehabilitation: Whose goals? Whose priorities? *Archives of Physical Medicine and Rehabilitation*, 1971b, **52**, 284-87.

Kutner, N., and Kutner, M. Race and sex as variables affecting reactions to disability. *Archives of Physical Medicine and Rehabilitation*, 1979, **60**, 62-66.

Lacerda, D. Behavior of quadriplegic patients and the hospital environment. Doctoral dissertation, University of Houston, 1970.

Landau, M. Body image in paraplegia: As a variable in adjustment to physical handicap. Doctoral dissertation, Columbia University, 1960.

Lane, J., and Barry, J. Recent research on client motivation. *Rehabilitation Research and Practice Review,* 1970, **1,** 5-25.

Lapatra, J. *Health care delivery systems: Evaluation criteria.* Springfield, Ill.: Charles C. Thomas, 1975.

Lawson, N. Depression after spinal cord injury: A multi-measure longitudinal study. Doctoral dissertation, University of Houston, 1976.

Lawson, N. Significant events in a rehabilitation center: A multilevel longitudinal approach. Paper presented at the American Congress of Rehabilitation Medicine, Miami Beach, October 1977.

Lawson, N. Significant events in the rehabilitation process: The spinal cord patients' point of view. *Archives of Physical Medicine and Rehabilitation,* 1978, **59,** 573-79.

Lazarus, A. Learning theory and the treatment of depression. *Behavior Research and Therapy,* 1968, **6,** 83-89.

Lefcourt, H. Internal versus external control of reinforcement: A review. *Psychological Bulletin,* 1966, **65,** 206-20.

Lefcourt, H. *Locus of control: Current trends in theory and research.* New York: John Wiley and Sons, 1976.

Levinson, D.; Darrow, C.; Klein, E.; Levinson, M.; and McKee, B. *The seasons of a man's life.* New York: Alfred A. Knopf, 1978.

Leviton, G. Professional and client viewpoints on rehabilitation issues. *Rehabilitation Psychology,* 1973, **20** (1).

Lindner, H. Perceptual sensitization to sexual phenomena in the chronic physically handicapped. *Journal of Clinical Psychology,* 1953, **9,** 67-68.

Litman, T. The influence of self conception and life orientation factors in the rehabilitation of the orthopedically disabled. *Journal of Health and Human Behavior,* 1962, **3,** 249-57.

Litman, T. An analysis of the sociological factors affecting the rehabilitation of physically handicapped patients. *Archives of Physical Medicine and Rehabilitation,* 1964, **45,** 9-16.

Little, N., and Stewart, L. Vocational rehabilitation of spinal cord injured individuals. *Selected research topics in spinal cord injury rehabilitation.* Grant no. 16-P-56813/6-13, Houston, Texas: Texas Institute for Rehabilitation and Research, July 1975.

Loeber, R. Engineering the behavioral engineer. *Annual Review of Behavior Therapy,* 1973, **1,** 765-76.

LoPiccolo, J., and Steger, J. The sexual interaction inventory: A new instrument for assessment of sexual dysfunction. *Archives of Sexual Behavior,* 1974, **3,** 585-95.

Lovitt, R. Sexual adjustment of spinal cord injury patients. *Rehabilitation Research and Practice Review,* 1970, **1,** 25-29.

Lowry, R. A group training program for families of spinal cord injured patients. *Proceedings of the 11th Veterans Administration Spinal Cord Injury Conference,* 1964, **11,** 223-24.

Ludwig, E., and Adams, S. Patient cooperation in a rehabilitation center: Assumption of the client role. *Journal of Health and Social Behavior,* 1968, **9,** 328-36.

Ludwig, E., and Collette, J. Disability, dependency, and conjugal roles. *Journal of Marriage and the Family,* 1969, **31,** 736-39.

Lynch, W. Recreation role in a rehabilitation center. *Rehabilitation Record,* 1972, **13,** 18-19.

McDaniel, J. *Physical disability and human behavior.* 2nd ed. New York: Pergamon Press, 1976.

McDaniel, J., and Sexton, A. Psychoendocrine studies of patients with spinal cord lesions. *Journal of Abnormal Psychology,* 1970, **76,** 117-22.

Maki, R.; Winograd, M.; and Hinkle, E. Counseling/psychotherapy approach in rehabilitation of a spinal cord injury population. *Archives of Physical Medicine and Rehabilitation,* 1976, **57,** 548, abstract.

Malament, I.; Dunn, M.; and Davis, R. Pressure sores: An operant conditioning approach to prevention. *Archives of Physical Medicine and Rehabilitation,* 1975, **56,** 161-65.

Manley, S. A definitive approach to group counseling. *Journal of Rehabilitation,* 1973, **39,** 38-40.

Manley, S., and Armstrong, M. A transitional living experience for the severely disabled. *Rehabilitation Counseling Bulletin,* 1976, **19,** 551-55.

Mann, W.; Godfrey, M.; and Dowd, E. The use of group counseling procedures in the rehabilitation of spinal cord injured patients. *American Journal of Occupational Therapy,* 1973, **27,** 73-77.

Manson, M. The measurement of intelligence of 102 male paraplegics. *Journal of Consulting Psychology,* 1950, **14,** 193-96.

Margolin, R. Motivational problems and resolutions in the rehabilitation of paraplegics and quadriplegics. *American Archives of Rehabilitation Therapy,* 1971, **20,** 94-103.

Marr, J.; Greenwood, R.; and Roessler, R. Personal communication, April 29, 1977.

Masters, W., and Johnson, V. *Human sexual response.* Boston: Little, Brown and Company, 1966.

Matlack, D. *Cost-effectiveness of spinal cord injury center treatment.* National Paraplegia Foundation, Chicago, Ill., October, 1974.

Medved, M., and Wallechinsky, D. *What really happened to the class of '65?* New York: Ballantine Books, 1976.

Meichenbaum, D. *Cognitive-behavior modification: An integrative approach.* New York: Plenum Press, 1977.

Mesch, J. Content analysis of verbal communication between spinal cord injured and nondisabled male college students. *Archives of Physical Medicine and Rehabilitation,* 1976, **57,** 25-30.

Meyerson, H. Sense of competence in the spinal cord injured. Doctoral dissertation, University of Houston, 1968.

Michael, J. Rehabilitation. In C. Neuringer and J. Michael (Eds.), *Behavior modification in clinical psychology.* New York: Appleton-Century-Crofts, 1970.

Mikulic, M. Reinforcement of independent and dependent patient behaviors by nursing personnel: An exploratory study. *Nursing Research,* 1971, **20,** 162-64.

Miller, D. Sexual counseling with spinal cord injured clients. *Journal of Sexual and Marital Therapy,* 1975, **1,** 312-18.

Miller, D.; Wolfe, M.; and Spiegel, M. Therapeutic groups for patients with spinal cord injuries. *Archives of Physical Medicine and Rehabilitation,* 1975, **56,** 130-35.

Miller, R., and Keith, R. A. Behavioral mapping in a rehabilitation hospital. *Rehabilitation Psychology,* 1973, **20,** 148-55.

Mitchell, K. The body image barrier variable and level of adjustment to stress induced by severe physical disability. *Journal of Clinical Psychology,* 1970, **26,** 49-52.

Money, J. Phantom orgasm in the dreams of paraplegic men and women. *Archives of General Psychiatry,* 1960a, **3,** 373-82.

Money, J. Components of eroticism in man: Cognitional rehearsals. In J. Wortis (Ed.), *Recent advances in biological psychiatry.* New York: Grune and Stratton, 1960b.

Mooney, T.; Cole, T.; and Chilgren, R. *Sexual options for paraplegics and quadriplegics.* Boston: Little, Brown and Company, 1975.

Moos, R. *Evaluating treatment environments: A social ecological approach.* New York: John Wiley and Sons, 1974.

Moos, R. *The human context: Environmental determinants of behavior.* New York: John Wiley and Sons, 1976.

Morgan, E.; Hohmann, G.; and Davis, J. Psychosocial rehabilitation in VA spinal cord injury centers. *Rehabilitation Psychology,* 1974, **21,** 3-33.

Mueller, A. Psychologic factors in rehabilitation of paraplegic patients. *Archives of Physical Medicine and Rehabilitation,* 1962a, **43,** 151-59.

Mueller, A. Pain study of paraplegic patients: The Rorschach test as an aid in predicting pain relief by means of chordotomy. *Archives of Neurology,* 1962b, **7,** 355-58.

Munro, D. The rehabilitation of patients totally paralyzed below the waist, with special reference to making them ambulatory and capable of earning their own living: V. An end result of study of 445 cases. *New England Journal of Medicine,* 1954, **250,** 4-14.

Nagler, B. Psychiatric aspects of cord injury. *American Journal of Psychiatry,* 1950, **107,** 49-56.

National spinal cord injury model systems conference: Proceedings. Phoenix, Ariz.: National Spinal Cord Injury Data Research Center, 1978.

Neff, W. Rehabilitation and work. In W. Neff (Ed.), *Rehabilitation Psychology.* Washington, D.C.: American Psychological Association, 1971.

Nichols, J. *Men's liberation: A new definition of masculinity.* New York: Penguin Books, 1975.

Nickerson, E. Some correlates of adjustment by paraplegics. *Perceptual and Motor Skills,* 1971, **32,** 11-23.

Norris-Baker, C. Negotiability in the home environments of persons with spinal cord injuries. Paper presented at the Southwestern Psychological Association, New Orleans, April 1978.

Nyquist, R., and Bors, E. Mortality and survival in traumatic myelopathy during 19 years from 1946-1965. *International Journal of Paraplegia,* 1967, **5,** 22-48.

O'Connor, J., and Leitner, L. Traumatic quadriplegia: A comprehensive review. *Journal of Rehabilitation,* 1971, **37,** 14-20.

Pigott, R. Behavior modification and control in rehabilitation. *Journal of Rehabilitation,* 1969, **35,** 12-15.

Pomerleau, O.; Bobrove, P.; and Smith, R. Rewarding psychiatric aides for the behavioral improvement of assigned patients, *Journal of Applied Behavior Analysis,* 1973, **6,** 383-90.

Pommer, D. and Streedbeck, D. Motivating staff performance in an operant learning program for children. *Journal of Applied Behavior Analysis,* 1974, **7,** 217-21.

Poor, C. Vocational rehabilitation of persons with spinal cord injuries. *Rehabilitation Counseling Bulletin,* 1975, **18,** 264-71.

Poor, C.; Fletcher, C.; Thielges, J.; Gutknecht, M.; and Morgan, C. Vocational potential assessment. *Archives of Physical Medicine and Rehabilitation,* 1975, **56,** 33-36.

Price, M. Causes of death in 11 of 227 patients with traumatic spinal cord injury over a period of nine years. *International Journal of Paraplegia,* 1973, **11,** 217-20.

Professional conference on research issues in the psychological, social, and vocational adjustment in spinal cord injury. Easter Seal Society of Los Angeles County, Los Angeles, April 28-29, 1977.

Rabin, B. *The sensuous wheeler.* Santa Ana, Calif.: Joyce Publications, 1974.

Rabinowitz, H. Motivation for recovery; Four social psychological aspects. *Archives of Physical Medicine and Rehabilitation,* 1961, **42,** 799-807.

Rachman, S. *The effects of psychotherapy.* New York: Pergamon Press, 1971.

Rainwater, L. Some aspects of lower class sexual behavior. *Medical Aspects of Human Sexuality,* 1968, **2,** 15-25.

Rainwater, L. Marital sexuality in four cultures of poverty. In D. Marshall and R. Suggs (Eds.), *Human sexual behavior.* New York: Basic Books, 1971.

Rapier, J.; Adelson, R.; Carey, R.; and Croke, K. Changes in children's attitudes toward the physically handicapped. *Exceptional Children,* 1972, **39,** 219-23.

Reynales, B. How literature affects the public's image of the handicapped. *Paraplegia News,* 1976, **29** (331), 16-17.

Richardson, S. Research report: Handicap, appearance, and stigma. *Social Science and Medicine,* 1971, **5,** 621-28.

Richardson, S.; Goodman, N.; Hastorf, A.; and Dornsbusch, S. Cultural uniformity in reaction to physical disabilities. *American Sociological Review,* 1961, **26,** 241-47.

Richardson, S., and Royce, J. Race and physical handicap in children's preference for other children. *Child Development,* 1968, **39,** 467-80.

Robertiello, R. The myth of physical attractiveness. *Psychotherapy,* 1976, **13** (13), 54-55.

Roberts, A. Spinal cord injury: Some psychological considerations. *Minnesota Medicine,* 1972, **55,** 1115-17.

Roberts, A.; Dinsdale, S.; Matthews, R.; and Cole, T. Modifying persistent undesirable behavior in a medical setting. *Archives of Physical Medicine and Rehabilitation,* 1969, **50,** 147-53.

Roberts, E. Invited address to staff at Rancho Los Amigos Hospital, Downey, Calif., January 26, 1976.

Robinson, W. Sport and recreation for the mentally and physically handicapped. *Nursing Times,* 1973, **69,** 895-97.

Roessler, R.; Milligan, T.; and Ohlson, A. Personal adjustment training for the spinal cord injured. *Rehabilitation Counseling Bulletin,* 1976, **19,** 544-50.

Rohrer, K.; Adelman, B.; Talbert, D.; Gamble, J.; and Johnson, E. Spinal cord injured individuals and their families: An interdisciplinary group approach for education and adjustment (a pilot study). *Archives of Physical Medicine and Rehabilitation,* 1976, **57,** 559, abstract.

Romano, M. Sexuality and the disabled female. *Accent on Living* (Winter) 1973a, 27-34.

Romano, M. Sexual counseling in groups. *Journal of Sex Research,* 1973b, **9,** 69-78.

Romano, M. Social skills training with the newly handicapped. *Archives of Physical Medicine and Rehabilitation,* 1976, **57,** 302-3.

Romano, M. Personal communication, February 5, 1978.

Romano, M., and Lassiter, R. Sexual counseling with the spinal cord injured. *Archives of Physical Medicine and Rehabilitation,* 1972, **53,** 568-72.

Rosenberg, B., and Bensman, J. Sexual patterns in three ethnic subcultures of an American underclass. In A. Juhasz (Ed.), *Sexual development and behavior: Selected readings.* Homewood, Ill.: The Dorsey Press, 1973.

Rosenthal, A. Aftermath—A follow-up study of patients with myelopathy. *Archives of Physical Medicine and Rehabilitation,* 1966, **47,** 793-96.

Rosillo, R., and Fogel, M. Correlation of psychologic variables and progress in physical rehabilitation: IV. The relation of body image to success in physical rehabilitation. *Archives of Physical Medicine and Rehabilitation,* 1971, **52,** 182-86.

Rotter, J. Generalized expectancies for internal versus external control of reinforcement. *Psychological Monographs: General and Applied,* 1966, **80,** 1-28.

Rottkamp, B. A behavior modification approach to nursing therapeutics in body positioning of spinal cord injured patients. *Nursing Research,* 1976, **25,** 181-86.

Rushmer, R. *Humanizing health care: Alternative futures for medicine.* Cambridge, Mass.: MIT Press, 1975.

Rusk, H. *Specialized placement of quadriplegics and other severely disabled.* Final report to the Vocational Rehabilitation Administration, no. RD 509, New York University Medical Center, Institute of Rehabilitation Medicine, April 1963.

Sadlick, M., and Penta, F. Changing student nurse attitudes towards quadriplegics by use of television. *Medical and Biological Illustration,* 1975, **25,** 129-32.

Safilios-Rothschild, Constantina. *The sociology and social psychology of disability and rehabilitation.* New York: Random House, 1970.

Salhoot, J. Group strategies with the severely physically handicapped. In M. Seligman (Ed.), *Group counseling and group psychotherapy with rehabilitation clients.* Springfield, Ill.: Charles C. Thomas, 1977.

Sand, P., and Berni, R. An incentive contract for nursing home aides. *American Journal of Nursing,* 1974, **74,** 475-77.

Sand, P.; Fordyce, W.; and Fowler, R. Fluid intake behavior in patients with spinal cord injury: Prediction and modification. *Archives of Physical Medicine and Rehabilitation,* 1973, **54,** 254-62.

Sand, P.; Fordyce, W.; Trieschmann, R.; and Fowler, R. Behavior modification in the medical rehabilitation setting: Rationale and some applications. *Rehabilitation Research and Practice Review,* 1970, **1,** 11-24.

Schachter, S. *Emotion, obesity, and crime.* New York: Academic Press, 1971.

Schimel, J. Self esteem and sex. In L. Gross (Ed.), *Sexual behavior–current issues.* Flushing, N.Y.: Spectrum Publications, 1974.

Schlenoff, D. A theory of career development for the quadriplegic. *Journal of Applied Rehabilitation Counseling,* 1975, **6,** 3-13.

Schofield, W. *Psychotherapy: The purchase of friendship.* Englewood Cliffs, N.J.: Prentice-Hall, 1964.

Seeman, M., and Evans, J. Alienation and learning in a hospital setting. *American Sociological Review,* 1962, **27,** 774-82.

Seligman, M. *Helplessness: On depression, development, and death.* San Francisco: W. H. Freeman and Company, 1975.

Seybold, J. Rehabilitation and employment status report. *Paraplegia News,* 1976, **29** (330), 34-36.

Seymour, C. Personality and paralysis: I. Comparative adjustment of paraplegics and quadriplegics. *Archives of Physical Medicine and Rehabilitation,* 1955, **36,** 691-94.

Sheehy, G. *Passages: Predictable crises of adult life.* New York: Bantam Books, 1974, 1976.

Sheredos, S. Games for the severely disabled. *Bulletin of Prosthetic Research,* 1973, **10,** 130-37.

Shontz, F. Behavior settings may affect rehabilitation client. *Rehabilitation Record,* 1967, **8** (2), 37-40.

Shontz, F. Physical disability and personality. In W. Neff (Ed.), *Rehabilitation Psychology.* Washington, D. C.: American Psychological Association, 1971.

Siegel, M. Planning for employment for the quadriplegic. *Proceedings of the 17th Veterans Administration Spinal Cord Injury Conference,* 1969a, **18,** 230-33.

Siegel, M. Vocational potential of the quadriplegic. *Medical Clinics of North America,* 1969b, **53,** 713-18.

Siegel, M. Driver training, transportation and vocational adjustment of the handicapped in an urban setting. *Psychological Aspects of Disability,* March 1970, **17,** 9-10.

Siegel, M. Improving employment horizons for the severely disabled. In R. Pacinelli (Ed.), *Research utilization in rehabilitation facilities.* International Association of Rehabilitation Facilities, October 1971.

Siller, J. Psychological situation of the disabled with spinal cord injuries. *Rehabilitation Literature,* 1969, **30,** 290-96.

Silver, J., and Owens, E. Sexual problems in disorders of the nervous system: II. Psychological reactions. *British Medical Journal,* 1975, **3,** 532-34.

Singh, S., and Magner, T. Sex and self: The spinal cord injured. *Rehabilitation Literature,* 1975, **36,** 2-10.

Skipper, J.; Fink, S.; and Hallenbeck, P. Physical disability among married women: Problems in the husband-wife relationship. *Journal of Rehabilitation,* 1968, **34,** 16-19.

Steger, J., and Brockway, J. Sexual enhancement in spinal cord injury patients: Behavioral group treatment. Paper presented at American Congress of Rehabilitation Medicine, New Orleans, November 1978.

Stock, D., and Cole, J. *Cooperative living: A cooperative self-support system for severely physically disabled young adults.* Final report of RSA. Grant no. 13-P-55487/6-01, Houston, Texas: Texas Institute for Rehabilitation and Research, 1977.

Swenson, E. The relationship between locus of control expectancy and successful rehabilitation of the spinal cord injured. Doctoral dissertation, Arizona State University, 1976.

Symington, D. and Fordyce, W. Changing concepts in the management of traumatic paraplegia. *General Practice,* 1965, **32** (3), 141-55.

Talbot, H. Psychosocial aspects of sexuality in spinal cord injury patients. *International Journal of Paraplegia*, 1971, **9**, 37-39.

Tanaka, T. Economic security for the disabled. Unpublished paper. Paramount City, Calif., 1977.

Taylor, D. Treatment goals for quadriplegic and paraplegic patients. *American Journal of Occupational Therapy*, 1974, **28**, 22-29.

Taylor, G. Predicted versus actual response to spinal cord injury: A psychological study. Doctoral dissertation, University of Minnesota, 1967.

Taylor, G. Moderator-variable effect on personality test item endorsements of physically disabled patients. *Journal of Consulting and Clinical Psychology*, 1970, **35**, 183-88.

Taylor, G., and Persons, R. Behavior modification techniques in a physical medicine and rehabilitation center. *Journal of Psychology*, 1970, **74**, 117-24.

Teal, J., and Athelstan, G. Sexuality and spinal cord injury: Some psychosocial considerations. *Archives of Physical Medicine and Rehabilitation*, 1975, **56**, 264-68.

Terkel, S. *Working*. New York: The Hearst Corporation, 1972 and 1974.

Tomita, C., and Matsubayashi, T. The effects of swimming for the severe spinal cord injuries. *International Journal of Paraplegia*, 1964, **3**, 88.

Tomko, M.; Griffith, E.; and Timms, R. Sexual adjustment counseling with the spinal cord injured male. *Journal of Applied Rehabilitation Counseling*, 1972, **3**, 167-72.

Trieschmann, R. *Living with a disability: A proposal for rehabilitation of the person with spinal injury*. Report of the Psychological, Social, and Vocational Input Conference, Southwest Regional System for Treatment of Spinal Injury, Phoenix, Arizona, February 25-26, 1971.

Trieschmann, R. Sex drives, sex acts, and sexuality. Paper presented at the American Congress of Rehabilitation Medicine, Washington, D.C., October 1973.

Trieschmann, R. Coping with a disability: A sliding scale of goals. *Archives of Physical Medicine and Rehabilitation*, 1974, **55**, 556-60.

Trieschmann, R. Systematic programming of the patient-treatment environment interaction. Paper presented at the American Association for the Advancement of Science, New York City, January 1975.

Trieschmann, R. Ecological influences on the motivation of the person with spinal injury. Paper presented at the American Congress of Rehabilitation Medicine, San Diego, November 1976.

Trieschmann, R. *The psychological, social, and vocational adjustment to spinal cord injury: A strategy for future research*. Final report and executive summary of Rehabilitation Services Administration. Grant no. 13-P-59011/9-01, Easter Seal Society of Los Angeles County, April 30, 1978a.

Trieschmann, R. The role of the psychologist in the treatment of spinal cord injury. *International Journal of Paraplegia*, 1978b, **16**, 212-19.

Trieschmann, R., and Sand, P. WAIS and MMPI correlates of increasing renal failure in adult medical patients. *Psychological Reports*, 1971, **29**, 1251-62.

Trieschmann, R.; Stolov, W.; and Montgomery, E. An approach to the treatment of abnormal ambulation resulting from conversion reaction. *Archives of Physical Medicine and Rehabilitation*, 1970, **51**, 198-206.

Trieschmann, R., and Willems, E. Programs for the physically disabled. In D. Glenwick and L. Jason (Eds.), *Behavioral community psychology: Progress and prospects*. Praeger, Inc., 1980, in press.

Trombly, C. Principles of operant conditioning related to orthotic training of quadriplegic patients. *American Journal of Occupational Therapy*, 1966, **20**, 217-20.

Trotter, A., and Inman, D. The use of positive reinforcement in physical therapy. *Physical Therapy*, 1968, **48**, 347-52.

Udin, H., and Keith, R. Patients' daily activities after discharge from a rehabilitation hospital. Paper presented at American Congress of Rehabilitation Medicine, New Orleans, November 1978.

Valens, E. *A long way up: The story of Jill Kinmont*. New York: Harper and Row, 1966.

Vash, C. The psychology of disability. *Rehabilitation Psychology,* 1975, **22,** 145-62.

Vineberg, S., and Willems, E. Observation and analysis of patient behavior in the rehabilitation hospital. *Archives of Physical Medicine and Rehabilitation,* 1971, **52,** 8-14.

Vista Hill Psychiatric Foundation drug abuse and alcoholism newsletter, January 1974 **2** (9).

Wachs, H., and Zaks, M. Studies of body image in men with spinal cord injury. *Journal of Nervous and Mental Disease,* 1960, **131,** 121-27.

Walker, R. Vocational rehabilitation of the quadriplegic. *Archives of Physical Medicine and Rehabilitation,* 1961, **42,** 716-21.

Walls, R. A reinforcement contingency analysis of rehabilitation. *Rehabilitation Research and Practice Review,* 1971, **2** (4), 29-35.

Webb, E.; Campbell, D.; Schwartz, R.; and Sechrest, L. *Unobtrusive measures: Nonreactive research in the social sciences.* Chicago: Rand McNally College Publishing Co., 1966.

Weiss, A., and Diamond, M. Sexual adjustment, identification, and attitudes of patients with myelopathy. *Archives of Physical Medicine and Rehabilitation,* 1966, **47,** 245-50.

Weissman, B., and Kutner, B. Role disorders in extended hospitalization. *Hospital Administration,* 1967, **12** (1), 52-59.

Welch, M., and Gist, J. *The open token economy system: A handbook for a behavioral approach to rehabilitation.* Springfield, Ill.: Charles C. Thomas, 1974.

Wendland, L. The measuring of patient cooperativeness. *Rehabilitation Psychology,* 1973, **20,** 121-25.

Widmer, M. The telephone interview as an approach to longitudinal behavior assessment in the community. Paper presented at the Southwestern Psychological Association, New Orleans, April 1978.

Wilcox, N., and Stauffer, E. Follow-up of 423 consecutive patients admitted to the spinal cord center, Rancho Los Amigos Hospital, 1 January to 31 December 1967. *International Journal of Paraplegia,* 1972, **10,** 115-22.

Willems, E. Interface of the hospital environment and patient behavior. *Archives of Physical Medicine and Rehabilitation,* 1972, **53,** 115-22.

Willems, E. *Longitudinal analysis of patient behavior.* Annual report of research activity, Texas Institute for Rehabilitation and Research, Houston, Texas, June 1975.

Willems, E. Behavioral ecology, health status, and health care: Applications to the rehabilitation setting. In I. Altman and J. Wohlwill (Eds.), *Human behavior and environment.* New York: Plenum Publishing Corp., 1976a.

Willems, E. Longitudinal analysis of patient behavior. Annual report of research activity, Texas Institute for Rehabilitation and Research, Houston, Texas, June 1976b.

Willems, E., and Vineberg, S. Direct observation of patients: The interface of environment and behavior. *Psychological Aspects of Disability,* 1969, **16,** 74-88.

Wilson, W. *A study of quadriplegics in employment.* Woodrow Wilson Rehabilitation Center, Fisherville, Va., 1972.

Wittkower, E.; Gingras, G.; Mergler, L.; Wigdor, B.; and Lepine, A. A combined psychosocial study of spinal cord lesions. *Canadian Medical Association Journal,* 1954, **71,** 109-15.

Wittreich, W., and Radcliffe, K. The influence of simulated mutilation upon the perception of the human figure. *Journal of Abnormal and Social Psychology,* 1955, **51,** 493-95.

Wortman, C., and Brehm, J. Responses to uncontrollable outcomes: An integration of reactance theory and the learned helplessness model. *Advances in Experimental Social Psychology,* 1975, **8,** 277-337.

Wright, B. *Physical disability—a psychological approach.* New York: Harper and Row, 1960.

Young, J. Personal communication, September 22, 1977.

Young, J. Personal communication, April 6, 1978.

Zubek, J. (Ed.) *Sensory deprivation: Fifteen years of research.* New York: Appleton-Century-Crofts, 1969.

Index

Activities of daily living (ADL), 4, 5-6, 12-13, 20, 23-24, 29-30, 78-79, 86, 113, 156, 157, 169, 185, 193, 194, 197, 200, 209-210, 211, 212

Adjustment, 3-4, 43, 44, 47, 51-52, 56, 60, 67, 69, 70, 71, 75-79, 83-85, 93, 99, 100, 102, 104, 110, 113, 118, 181, 190, 193, 195, 197, 213

process of, 4, 35, 44, 54, 66, 88, 102-103, 148, 178

stages of, 37, 43-44, 45-46, 46-47, 83, 179, 206-207

Age, 22, 36, 58, 74, 75, 77, 78-79, 85, 93, 96, 98-100, 110, 115, 118-19, 137, 181, 184

Age of onset, 3, 15-19, 36, 78, 98-100, 113, 137, 181

Aging, 109-110

Alcohol, 21, 69, 75, 84, 180

Attitudes, 19, 60, 87, 88-89, 90, 91, 93, 110, 175, 183-84

of employers, 19, 120, 122, 126, 183, 191

of rehabilitation staff, 70-73, 84, 142, 150, 153, 181

Behavioral mapping, 148, 199-200

Behavior therapy, 161-66, 180, 185, 194, 198

Biochemical measures of emotion, 53-54, 179, 197-98, 206

Bladder and bowel function, 4, 8, 10, 11, 12, 19, 22, 24, 29, 71, 72, 94, 119, 129, 130, 156, 209

Body image, 38-39, 65-67, 84, 180

Case manager approach, 174, 185, 207

Chemotherapy, 10, 41, 42, 69, 83, 170-71, 179

Cooperation, 26, 37, 51, 57-59, 72, 73, 76, 77-78, 114, 195, 196

Cooperative living center, 173, 207

Counseling, 26, 28, 29, 40, 68, 140-41, 145, 157-161, 168, 184-85

Culture-ethnic group, 17, 63, 75, 86, 93, 97, 104, 138-39, 181

Decubitus ulcers, 7, 21, 29, 68, 78, 79-81, 101, 156, 157, 164, 209

Denial, 38, 42, 43-44, 45, 46, 47, 48, 51-52, 56, 83, 94, 179

Depression, 20, 24, 29-30, 37, 43-45, 47-53, 55-56, 59, 63, 65, 70-71, 72, 74, 75, 77, 81, 83-84, 101, 104, 137, 170-71, 179-180, 181-82, 195, 197-98

Devaluation, 3, 19, 43, 46, 88, 91-92, 106, 166

Divorce, 18, 92, 95-98, 141, 183

Drug abuse, 21, 68-69, 75, 84, 180

Duration of disability, 21, 22, 36, 98, 102-103, 110, 181

Education, 18-19, 20, 23, 63, 75-76, 96, 98, 104, 114, 115-16, 117-120, 126, 172, 181, 183

Ejaculation, 9, 133

Emotional reaction to disability, 22, 38, 44-45, 48, 51-54, 68, 75, 112-126, 179, 206

Employment, 19, 51, 63, 76, 77, 79, 95-97, 98, 112-126, 183, 190, 192

Erection, 8-9, 133, 137

Family, 3, 10, 13, 29-30, 40, 42, 48, 49, 59, 76-77, 78, 79, 85, 86-87, 92-98, 110, 113, 119, 144, 149, 156, 158, 181, 183, 193, 208

Fertility, 8, 9, 133

Financial disincentives, 19, 120-23, 124-25, 126, 181, 183, 191, 207
Financial resources, 14, 22, 36, 38, 76, 78, 79, 85, 94, 97, 104, 110, 121

Homebound rehabilitation programs, 174, 185, 207

Independence, 5-6, 19, 58, 72, 73, 79, 99, 109, 136, 149-150, 151-52, 154, 156, 163, 170, 172-73, 184, 200, 209
Independent living centers, 108, 175-176, 185, 207
Intelligence, 22, 81, 201

Learned helplessness, 50, 60-62, 64, 84, 153-54, 180
Learning
  process of, 20, 64, 147
  principles of, 26, 59-60, 162, 165, 213
Learning model of rehabilitation, 23, 26-29, 81, 178, 185, 211
Leisure, 3, 19, 30, 172, 183, 208
  See also Recreation
Level of injury, 4, 8-9, 14-15, 21, 22, 68, 77, 78, 80, 81, 92, 98-99, 100-102, 114, 116, 129-130, 132, 133, 145
  Cervical, 4-5, 8, 10-11, 12, 14, 40, 41, 42, 51, 52, 54, 63, 72, 94, 100, 115
  Lumbar, 4, 6, 8, 9, 12, 54
  Sacral, 4, 6, 8, 9, 12, 68
  Thoracic, 4, 6, 8, 10-11, 54
Locus of control, 50-51, 53, 57, 61-64, 75, 80, 83, 84, 100, 101, 104, 120, 153-54, 180, 181, 193, 201, 207
Longitudinal Functional Assessment System (LFAS), 190, 203-206

Marriage, 18, 21, 22, 75, 93, 95-98, 105, 144, 145, 183, 184, 208
Medical model of rehabilitation, 23, 24-29, 81, 178, 185
Medication, 10, 41, 42, 69, 83, 170-71, 179
Mobility, 6, 12-13, 20, 23-24, 29, 71, 86, 113, 156, 157, 169, 185, 193, 194, 197, 200, 209-210, 211, 212

Modeling, 106, 167-68, 175-76
Motivation, 24, 26, 28-29, 41, 57-61, 63-65, 72, 84, 119, 151-53, 154, 180, 185
  treatment of, 28, 29, 59-60, 84
Mourning, 43-44, 56, 57, 59, 60, 179
Multistage rehabilitation, 169, 184-85, 207, 209-212

National Spinal Cord Injury Data Research Center, 15, 196, 202

Pain, 7, 9-10, 38, 39, 42, 66, 68-70, 83, 84, 179, 180, 196
Peer counseling, 108, 175
Penile prostheses, 144-45
Personality, 46, 47, 48, 55, 63, 64, 65, 66, 70, 73-76, 79-81, 82-83, 99, 123, 181
Phantom orgasm, 8-9, 131-32, 134
Phantom sensations, 65-66, 68
Physical attractiveness, 67, 87, 89-90, 136, 182
Preinjury history, 69, 73, 73-75, 77-79, 93, 98, 118-120, 141, 191, 208
Pressure sores, 7, 21, 29, 68, 78, 79-81, 101, 156, 157, 164, 209
Productivity, 29, 77, 85, 93, 99, 101, 112-126, 138, 183, 185, 193, 199, 201, 206, 207, 208
Psychopathology, 29, 49, 59, 75, 181
Psychosis, 43, 47, 48, 75
Psychotherapy, 26, 28, 29, 57, 84, 157-161, 168, 184

Recreation, 19, 23, 30, 72, 108-109, 149, 183, 193, 208
  See also Leisure
Regional Model Spinal Cord Injury Treatment System, 13-14, 15
Rehabilitation, definition of, 20, 26, 60, 156, 212
  learning model of, 23, 26-29, 81, 178, 185, 211
  medical model of, 23, 24-29, 81, 178, 185
Rehabilitation Indicators Project (RIP), 190, 203, 204, 206

About the Author

Roberta B. Trieschmann (Ph. D., University of Minnesota) is Director of Psychological Services at St. Jude Hospital and Rehabilitation Center in Fullerton, California. Her primary interest is the integration of psychosocial services with medical rehabilitation and the application of behavioral technologies to the problems of health care and physical disability.

She has been on the faculties of the University of Washington and the University of Cincinnati and initiated the program of psychological services at the first regional model spinal injury treatment center which is located in Phoenix, Arizona. She is a member of the American Psychological Association, the American Congress of Rehabilitation Medicine, and the International Medical Society of Paraplegia, and has been listed in *Who's Who of American Women* since 1975.

Dr. Trieschmann is the author or coauthor of over 20 publications in scientific journals or books. She has served as a consultant to rehabilitation centers and organizations nationally and internationally in regard to psychosocial issues of physical disability and the delivery of rehabilitation services. Currently she is on the editorial board of *Rehabilitation Psychology*.

Pergamon General Psychology Series

Editors: Arnold P. Goldstein, Syracuse University
Leonard Krasner, SUNY, Stony Brook

Date Due

OCT 3 0 1981		JUL 7 1982
FEB 6 1982		FEB 2 1 1989
NOV 1 5 1984		MAR 2 1 1989
DEC 2 2 1984		MAY 15 1989
MAR 2 3 1985 MAR 1 9 1986		MAY 0 9 1990 #5931780
MAY 2 7 1988		
		AUG 0 8 1995
		JUN 1 4 1996 AUG 0 5 1998 MAR 1 9 1999